PFO AND THE DIVER

PATENCY OF CARDIAC FORAMEN OVALE A RISK FACTOR FOR DYSBARIC DISORDERS?

PFO AND THE DIVER

PATENCY OF CARDIAC FORAMEN OVALE
A RISK FACTOR FOR DYSBARIC DISORDERS?

CONSTANTINO BALESTRA

FRANS J. CRONJÉ

PETER GERMONPRÉ

ALESSANDRO MARRONI

DAN EUROPE REASEARCH DIVISION
DIVING SAFETY LABORATORY
ENVIRONMENTAL AND OCCUPATIONAL PHYSIOLOGY DEPARTMENT
(Haute Ecole Paul Henri Spaak)
UNIVERSITE LIBRE DE BRUXELLES
CENTER FOR HYPERBARIC OXYGEN THERAPY BRUSSELS
DAN SOUTH AFRICA

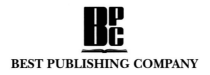

BEST PUBLISHING COMPANY

Design: Bill Owen
        Kelly Phillips
        Travis Moore

Edited By: James T. Joiner
            Kate Lasky

No responsibility is assumed by the Publisher or Editors for any injury and/or damage to persons or property as a matter of product liability, negligence or otherwise, or from any use or operation of any methods, product, instructions or ideas contained in the material herein. No suggested test or procedure should be carried out unless, in the reader's judgement, its risk is justified. Because of rapid advances in the medical sciences, we recommend that the independent verifications of diagnoses and drug dosages are the responsibilities of the reader.

Copyright © 2007 by Best Publishing Company

International Standard Book Number-13:978-1-930536-39-5
International Standard Book Number-10:1-930536-39-9
Library of Congress Control Number: 2007927234

For more information contact:
Best Publishing Company
2355 North Steves Boulevard
P.O. Box 30100
Flagstaff, AZ 86003-0100 USA

Tele: 928.527.1055
Fax: 928.526.0370
divebooks@bestpub.com
www.bestpub.com

CONTENTS

SECTION 3. REFERENCES

ACKNOWLEDGEMENTS

Upon completion of any large project, it is a challenge to thank all those who have contributed without inadvertently omitting someone. As such, the authors apologize in advance for any accidental omissions.

Many have contributed through discussions and ideas and in this we would like to thank: Prof. Peter Bennett, Prof. David Elliott, Prof. Alf Brubakk, Prof. Philip James, Dr. Bernard Gardette, Dr. Daniel Carturan, Dr. Stéphane Besnard, Dr. Daniel Slosman, Dr. Hans Ornhagen, Dr. Greta Bolstadt, Prof. Francis Wattel, Prof. Daniel Mathieu and others

Others, more closely associated with the project—at least geographically—include: Prof. Jacques Duchateau, Prof. Karl Hainaut, Dr. Brigitte Farkas, Frédéric Vanderschueren, Dr. Paul Dendale, Prof. Guy Cheron, Dr. Philippe Unger, Dr. Guy Vandenhoven, Dr. Jean-Claude Lemper, Jean Pierre Imbert, Thyl Snoeck, Mikel Ezquer, Dr. Jordi Desola, Dr. Juerg Wendling, Dr. Adel Taher, Dr. Ulrich Van Laak, Dr. Ole Hyldegaard, Dr. Ramiro Cali-Corleo, Dr. Francis Hastir, Dr. Stefaan Deneweth, Dr. Herman Van Bogaert, Prof. Jacques Poortmans, Prof. Philippe Van de Borne, Prof. Robert Naeije, Petra Jerabkova, Oldrich Zmeskal, Jan Haderka and others we may have omitted accidentally!

Special thanks to our former students Nicolas Seget for the wonderful anatomical drawings. We wish to thank all of you for your invaluable support.

PREFACE

This is a book directed towards meeting the needs of those who wish to study the fuller picture of a current issue and gain a wider view of relevant opinions. There will always be limits to the rate of spreading new lessons learned from recent research because of the lengthy processes of publishing peer-reviewed papers, of other persons then assessing those findings and finally of applying them to new research or possibly direct to practical applications.

This delay is nothing new. Nearly a hundred years ago, in a book largely about decompression from compressed air,[1] Sir Leonard Hill despaired of the many "astounding hypotheses" that were confusing this topic and he particularly deplored the slowness of many around the world to accept "the magnificent work of the French school." He was, of course, referring to Paul Bert's review of his extensive researches.[2] These were still not yet recognized as the foundation of hyperbaric medicine even though Bert's work had been published more than 30 years previously.

Today electronic publication of peer-reviewed papers may seem to have shortened the latency for the dissemination of new scientific work but while some discussion may be available through the world wide web, there are still limits on accessibility to publications by those who are interested in keeping abreast of developments. Thus a broad overview of their various researches by a particular group can facilitate assessment of otherwise seemingly unconnected papers and can catalyse new thoughts before the investigators run out of money or momentum. Not everything discussed in this particular overview will be sustained as correct but what is more important is that it grasps the breadth and complexity of some developments in decompression safety that are relatively recent.

Within the range of distinct pathologies associated with decompression, there are a number of other clinically-related conditions, such as pulmonary barotrauma (PB), that are not directly relevant to the possible role of a PFO. Although the clinical presentations of their emboli may be very similar, only passing references are needed here to arterial gas embolism (AGE) which is from the traumatic intravasation of alveolar gas and its direct passage as bubbles from the pulmonary veins into the systemic arteries. This type of bubble embolism can of course occur when the regional tissues are already loaded with dissolved gas and this can lead to a biphasic presentation that combines features of AGE and DCS sequentially.[3] Because AGE is not the result of a right-to-left cardiac shunt of venous bubbles, PB and AGE are beyond the immediate relevance of this book. The focus here is on PFO as a risk factor and thus the text is concerned primarily with dissolved gas and the subsequent aberrant distribution of those venous bubbles in the presence of a natural and common anatomical variant of cardiac development.

David H Elliott O.B.E.
D.Phil., F.RC.P., F.F.O.M.

---

[1] Hill L. Caisson Sickness and the Physiology of Work in Compressed Air. London: Arnold. 1912.

[2] Bert P. La pression barométrique. Recherches de physiologie expérimentale. 1878. Hitchcock MA, Hitchcock FA, translators. Undersea Medical Society: Bethesda, Maryland. 1978.

[3] Neuman TS Arterial gas embolism and pulmonary barotrauma. Pp 557-577 in Bennett and Elliott's Physiology and Medicine of Diving. 5th edition. Brubakk AO & Neuman TS (Eds). Saunders: Edinburgh. 2003.

DEDICATION

Adrien
Ambre
Faye
Flores
Francesca
Laura
Marine
Renée
and
Millicent

and all those who may yet be added in the years to come...

...also to our wives Anne-Marie, Elke, Nuccia, and Lucie ...for adding them.

DISCLAIMER

The views expressed by the authors are their own and do not necessarily reflect the opinion of the doctors, Divers Alert Network(DAN), or Best Publishing Company.

While the information in this book is consistent with good medical practice, no responsibility can be assumed by the author or the publisher for any injuries or damage of any nature whatsoever, as a result of product failure, negligence, or from the application of any recommendations or ideas contained in this book.

Medicine is an ever-changing field. Standard safety precaution must be followed, but as new research and clinical experience broaden our knowledge, changes in treatment and drug therapy may become necessary or appropriate. Readers are advised to check the most current product information provided by the manufacturer of each drug, device, or equipment to verify the recommended dose, the method and duration of administration, and contraindications.

Section 1
An Introduction to Clinical Aspects of Decompression Illness Dysbaric Disorders

CHAPTER 1

AN INTRODUCTION TO CLINICAL ASPECTS OF DECOMPRESSION ILLNESS (DCI)/DYSBARIC DISORDERS

INTRODUCTION

Decompression Illness (DCI)/Dysbaric disorders represent a complex spectrum of pathophysiological conditions with a wide variety of signs and symptoms related to dissolved gas and its subsequent phase change.

Any significant organic or functional decrement in individuals who have recently been exposed to a reduction in environmental pressure (i.e., decompression) must be considered as possibly having DCI until proven otherwise. However, apart from the more obvious acute manifestations, individuals who have experienced repetitive exposures (e.g., commercial or professional divers and active recreational divers) may also develop sub-acute or chronic manifestations—sub-clinically and insidiously. It is, in fact, generally accepted that sub-clinical forms of DCI exist, with little or no reported symptoms, and that these may cause changes in the bones, the central nervous system and the lungs (Kelemen, 1983; Shinoda et al., 1997; Wilmshurst and Ross, 1998).

Generally speaking, a *disorder* is a physical derangement, frequently slight and transitory in nature. On the other hand, a *disease* is considered a condition of an organ, part, structure or system of the body in which there is abnormal function resulting from genetic predisposition, diet or environmental factors. *Diseases* are typically more serious, active, prolonged and deep-rooted (Webster dictionary).

DCI should initially be considered a *disorder* due to a distinct physical cause, which can subsequently transform into a *disease* if adequate and timely action is not undertaken to abort or to minimize the pathophysiological effects of bubbles within body tissues.

The primary physical cause of DCI is the separation of gas in body tissues due to inadequate decompression leading to an excessive degree of gas super-saturation in the body tissues (Kumar et al., 1990). Rapid decompression (rate of ascent or omission of decompression stops) is a primary cause of gas separation in body tissues.

The most obvious prevention strategy for DCI is therefore determining and observing appropriate ascent and decompression procedures (Marroni and Zannini, 1981; Marroni et al., 2001b).

Unfortunately, the recommendations for decompression are not always reliable. This is confirmed by the finding that more than half the cases of DCI managed by Divers Alert Network (DAN) worldwide over the past several years have not been associated with an obvious violation of decompression procedures, dive tables or dive computer limits; they have been "unpredictable."

This has led to a search for other contributing factors to the development of DCI, such as a Patent Foramen Ovale, in an effort to explain a wide variation in individual susceptibility to DCI. Other contributing factors include complement activation in the presence of gas bubbles as well as various complex interactions between gas bubbles, blood cells, and the capillary endothelial lining.

The manifestations of DCI are sometimes transient, trivial or subtle. Accordingly, they are likely to be ignored or denied by individual divers, training organizations and emergency physicians unless these individuals are specifically educated and made aware of the manifestations of DCI. Importantly, however, not only are there growing concerns about under-reporting, under-estimation and under-treatment of DCI, but also that this may result in permanent organic or functional damage. Accordingly, it is important to raise the index of suspicion amongst divers and physicians alike.

One of the ongoing challenges regarding DCI prevention, detection and management is that there is no diagnostic test—no gold standard—to determine with any certainty that the plethora of possible clinical manifestations following decompression exposure are indeed related to bubbles. Over the past century, the closest surrogate has been a non-invasive indicator of decompression stress—precordial Doppler-detected venous gas bubbles, which appear typically within the first two hours after decompression.

Although the presence of Doppler-detectable gas bubbles in the blood is not necessarily predictive of clinically evident DCI, the appearance of DCI in the absence of detectable venous gas emboli (i.e., bubbles) is rare. There is even growing experimental and clinical evidence that suggests that asymptomatic "silent" bubbles in the body may be causing significant cellular

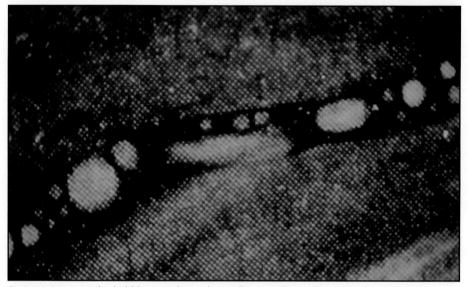

Figure 1. Intravascular bubbles in rodent sub maxillary capillaries (Courtesy of A. Marroni).

and biological reactions that release damaging biochemical substances in the blood. Accordingly, the threshold of concern is slowly moving away from the clinical reaction to bubbles (i.e., DCI) towards the appearance of bubbles themselves (i.e., venous gas emboli).

DEFINING DCI

The traditional classification of DCI—i.e. Type I or Type II Decompression Sickness (DCS) and Arterial Gas Embolism—is now considered inadequate for diagnostic and therefore for clinical management in that it is based on the specific underlying pathophysiology which is not always known at the time. We now know this not to be the case; indeed, there is also great disparity in the application of this classification of DCI between specialists when asked to define the same cases of dysbaric disorders. Consequently, a descriptive classification has appeared which uses the common term "DCI" or dysbarism, followed by a description of the clinical signs and symptoms, their onset and progression. The latter system has been considered both more universally understandable and simpler to teach. It also shows a much higher degree of concordance between the specialists describing the same DCI cases. For purposes of clarity and consistency, in the text DCI refers to dysbaric disorders that are clearly due to decompression sickness or where the origin of embolized gas cannot be attributed with certainty to arterial gas embolism due to pulmonary barotrauma. Where the cause of arterial embolization is the direct consequence of pulmonary overexpansion, the term arterial gas embolism (AGE) is used.

Epidemiologically, there is universal consensus among the international diving medicine community that the incidence of DCI is generally very low and that there is no significant gender-related susceptibility. There is also consensus that neurological manifestations are by far the most common form of DCI amongst recreational divers.

Many, as yet unknown aspects of DCI, are the object of ongoing international studies. These include the relationship between gas separation and DCI injury; the relationship between clinical symptoms and the severity of the disease; the relationship between initial clinical onset, treatment results and permanent *sequelae*; the reason for the large variation in individual susceptibility to DCI; the lifespan of gas bubbles; and the *true incidence* of DCI.

HISTORICAL PERSPECTIVES

In 1670, Robert Boyle demonstrated that DCI could be produced in a reptile by a sudden lowering of atmospheric pressure. The subsequent first clinical recording of DCI was in compressed air workers: In 1845, Triger reported that two men had suffered "very sharp pain" in the left arm while another had pain in the knees and left shoulder 30 minutes after emerging from a seven-hour exposure to between 2.4 atmospheres and 4.25 atmospheres of pressure. Although not knowing what it was, the first empirical clinical treatment for DCI was also reported by Triger—"rubbing with spirits of wine soon relieved this pain in both men and they kept working on the following days" (Triger, 1845). Some years later, Pol and Wattelle wrote that they were "justified in hoping that a sure and prompt means of relief would be to recompress immediately, then decompress very carefully" (Pol and Wattelle, 1854). Even so, it was only many years later that their advice was heeded.

In 1878, Paul Bert demonstrated that the cause of DCI was dissolved nitrogen going into gas phase in body tissues and that this bubble formation was responsible for its manifestations. Bert also highlighted the existence of "silent bubbles" in venous blood. He understood that recompression was the primary treatment and that it should be applied promptly. He also used oxygen at one atmosphere following very rapid decompression and observed that cardiopulmonary symptoms, but not spinal cord paralysis, could be relieved by normobaric oxygen breathing (Bert et al., 1943).

The *Journal of the Society of Art* of May 15, 1896 describes the work of Mr. E. W. Moir during the excavations of the tunnel under the Hudson River in 1889. Facing a tragic fatality rate of 25% of the workers due to DCI, he installed a recompression chamber at the work site. As a direct result of this intervention, there were only two further deaths over the following 15 months in the 120 workers involved with a project. Moir wrote:

> *"With a view to remedying the state of things an air compartment like a boiler was made in which the men could be treated homeopathically, or reimmersed in compressed air. It was erected near the top of the shaft, and when a man was overcome or paralyzed, as I have seen them often, completely unconscious and unable to use their limbs, they were carried into the compartment and the air pressure raised to about 1/2 or 2/3 of that in which they had been working, with immediate improvement. The pressure was then lowered at the very slow rate of one pound per minute or even less. The time allowed for equalization being from 25 to 30 minutes, and even in severe cases the men went away quite cured." (Moir, 1896)*

Unknowingly, Moir was recording both the means of preventing as well as treating DCI. Variations of his techniques—now called surface decompression—remain in use to this day.

Even though few subsequent publications appeared on recompression treatment for the next 30 years, it was a widely held notion that—to be effective— recompression should commence promptly followed by slow decompression. These principles remain in effect to this day even though the pressures, breathing gases and rates of decompression have changed significantly.

ETIOLOGY AND PATHOPHYSIOLOGY OF DCI

The clinical manifestations of DCI are protean. They follow the appearance of gas bubbles produced by a rapid lowering of ambient pressure. This pressure reduction causes dissolved inert gas to enter a gas phase causing the formation of gas bubbles in body tissues and fluids.

The clinical syndrome is known by many names including DCI, dysbaric illness, decompression sickness, decompression injury, caisson disease, bends, chokes, staggers, dysbarism and gas bubble injury.

Although arterial gas embolism is usually associated with pulmonary barotrauma, decompression bubbles (i.e., venous gas emboli) can become arterial (i.e., paradoxical gas embolism) if there is shunting between the venous and systemic circulation (e.g., intracardiac and intra-pulmonary shunting). This blurs the boundaries between decompression sickness and arterial gas embolism—which is why the term DCI was created.[†]

[†] Many languages are unable to differentiate between "sickness" and "illness" so that "dysbarism," "dysbaric illness" or "dysbaric injury" have become equivalent terms for DCI.

Clinical Settings of DCI[†]

Reduction in ambient pressure is not uniquely associated with diving. Several human activities involve regular or potential exposure to decompression:

- Diving
- Aviation
- Hyperbaric oxygen therapy (Nurses, Chamber assistants, Medical Personnel)
- Caisson Work and tunneling under pressure

Accordingly, under certain conditions, DCI may be associated with any of these activities.

Predisposing Factors

While a reduction in ambient pressure is the undisputed causal factor in DCI, the chances of developing DCI are greatly influenced by the pressure and duration of exposure; the subsequent rate of decompression; and a variety of additional factors that appear to increase individual susceptibility to DCI. For instance, exercise during exposure to increased ambient pressure (during the bottom phase of the dive) appears to increase the incidence of DCI significantly. The probable explanation is that exercise at pressure increases blood flow and therefore also the delivery of inert gas to tissues. This additional burden of inert gas needs to be eliminated during decompression to avoid DCI. Paradoxically, mild exercise during decompression stops may reduce susceptibility, whereas increased activity during pressure change again appears to increase the DCI risk. At least three mechanisms may help to explain the contradictory effects of exercise:

- The formation of gas micronuclei: Rapid or turbulent blood flow, especially where blood vessels divide, may create pockets of negative pressure due a Venturi effect. Inert gas, drawn into these areas by the pressure gradient, can form small gas collections called micronuclei. These seedling bubbles may then become the focal point, or nidus, for further bubble growth formation.
- Increased local CO_2 production in exercising muscle may also have an effect: CO_2 is a highly diffusible gas that may contribute to the formation of these gas micronuclei. Even small increases in inspired CO_2 seem to increase the incidence of DCI. The mechanism is not clearly understood.
- Increases in core body temperature, due to increased muscle activity, may reduce the solubility of gas in body tissues, which may lead to bubble formation.

Interestingly, very recent research results are casting doubts on some previous assumptions regarding exercise prior to diving. Traditional thinking has been that exercise prior to diving may increase micronuclei and subsequent

---

[†] For purposes of clarity and consistency, in the test DCI refers to dysbaric disorders that are clearly due to decompression sickness or where the origin of embolized gas cannot be attributed with certainty to arterial gas embolism due to pulmonary barotrauma. Where the cause of arterial embolization is the direct consequence of pulmonary overexpansion, the term arterial gas embolism (AGE) is used.

inert gas delivery to tissues due to the increase in blood flow. It now appears, under certain conditions that exercise approximately 20 to 24 hours prior to diving lowers DCI incidence. The explanation of these findings is still incomplete, although nitric oxide production and modified architecture of blood vessel linings (i.e., endothelium) seem to be involved (Wisloff and Brubakk, 2001; Wisloff et al., 2003; Dujic et al., 2004; Wisloff et al., 2004).

Several other risk factors have also been proposed: There is an association between recent local musculoskeletal injuries and an increased incidence of DCI at or near the site of the injury. The mechanisms responsible for this phenomenon are unclear but include proposed changes in local blood flow and increased gas micronuclei formation in injured tissue.

Diving in cold water appears to increase the incidence of DCI. Inert gas uptake is generally not affected initially since the diver is usually warm to begin with (Martini et al., 1989; Gerriets et al., 2000). However, the diver tends to cool during the dive and may even be hypothermic by the time they ascend and perform their safety/decompression stops. The reduced body temperature offers greater solubility to inert gas, whereas circulation, particularly to the skin, is significantly reduced in an effort to preserve heat. The net result is a greater retention of inert gas during that dive. As the diver rewarms after the dive, the excess gas may be released as bubbles.

Advancing age increases the incidence of DCI for reasons that are not yet clearly known.

Dehydration is associated with diving, and may be a risk factor for DCI due to fluid shifts and haemodynamic changes (Boussuges et al., 2006). Studies on high-altitude aviation during World War II support this. The exact mechanism remains unclear. Changes in surface tension of serum favoring bubble formation have been postulated. Anecdotal reports also suggest that alcohol ingestion prior to diving increases the incidence of DCI—possibly by a similar mechanism.

There is anecdotal evidence suggesting that significant fatigue prior to diving is also a risk factor for DCI. It is uncertain whether the fatigue is a subtle indicator of unidentified biochemical or unspecified hemodynamic factors.

Pathogenesis of DCI (DCI)

Vascular obstruction

The single most important element in the pathogenesis of DCI appears to be a vascular obstruction by bubbles or bubble-formed complexes. This may affect both systemic or the pulmonary circulatory systems. The obstruction may be due to an accumulation of bubbles entering the circulation from supersaturated tissues and slowing down venous return. Alternatively it may be due to embolization of vascular beds by bubbles formed elsewhere. The effects may be insignificant in non-critical areas such as fatty tissue, but may become life threatening in others such as the central nervous system and cardiopulmonary systems.

Generalized vascular obstruction leads to oxygen deficiency, metabolic acidosis and hypovolemia due to increased capillary leakage. The acidosis and hypovolemia may also impair cardiovascular function—compounding the effects.

Vascular obstruction of pulmonary capillaries, secondary to embolization of venous gas bubbles or bubble-formed complexes, leads to increased pulmonary vascular resistance, bronchiolar constriction and peribronchiolar edema. These changes may lead to an imbalance between ventilation and circulation (i.e., ventilation-perfusion mismatch) with arterial hypoxemia—the "chokes."

Blood-bubble interactions: coagulation

Much attention has been devoted to the possible consequences of blood-bubble interactions: Bubbles appear capable of activating Hageman Factor (Factor XII) by converting it to Factor XIIa, which provokes coagulation; this further contributes to vascular obstruction.

Bubbles constitute a foreign body in the blood so that the complement cascade (i.e., the mechanisms of immunity and inflammation) are also activated through Factor XIIa. The sequence of reactions of this system produces a series of factors that increase capillary leakage and attract white blood cells to the area. Factor XIIa is also capable of activating the Kinin-Bradykinin System with the release of bradykinin and histamine. Bradykinin may cause local pain while both are capable of further increasing capillary leakage.

Bubbles may even cause breakdown of blood fats (i.e., lipoproteins) with the release of large quantities of lipid. Electron-micrographic studies in animals have shown vascular obstruction by a complex which appears to be composed of a gas bubble surrounded by a layer of lipid, to which blood platelets are sticking. This and similar observations have prompted research on the use of anticoagulants in DCI. To date there is still no firm evidence that disseminated intravascular coagulation occurs in humans nor has routine anti-coagulation proven to be useful as a therapy. However, an increased clotting tendency in isolated tissue areas may contribute significantly to the pathogenesis of DCI and this is the origin of the historic recommendation to use aspirin in the treatment of DCI.

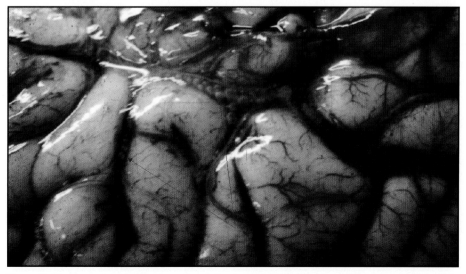

Figure 2. Massive gas embolism in a diver following fatal DCI (Courtesy of Dr. Yehuda Melamed, Israel)

Local versus vascular bubbles

There is little doubt that the localized pain in joints is the result of local gas formation.

Webb, et al. have demonstrated gas in periarticular and perivascular tissue spaces (Webb et al., 1944a; Webb et al., 1944b; Ferris and Engel, 1951). They have also successfully correlated the presence of gas with the occurrence of localized pain. The effectiveness of local pressure in relieving such pain—such as by inflating a blood pressure cuff—adds legitimacy to the hypothesis. Importantly, DCI frequently occurs simultaneously in several sites and there is a concern that overt limb pain may distract physicians from looking for subtle but more serious neurological abnormalities.

While bubbles within tissues are usually symptomatic, significant amounts of venous gas may be present without any clinical manifestations. In fact, incidental precordial Doppler detection of bubbles in the right ventricle or pulmonary arteries does not have significant positive predictive value for DCI. However, high degrees of bubbling are associated with an increased risk of developing symptoms. Conversely, Brubakk, et al. have never observed DCI symptoms in the absence of venous gas in the pulmonary artery and in the muscles of the thigh (Brubakk, 2003). They have argued that Doppler detection —which is performed at intervals—may occasionally miss bubbles and that the few exceptional cases who have presented with DCI symptoms but had no Doppler bubble signals, may have been false negatives. Similarly, Nishi has reported that DCI is always accompanied by bubbles if all monitoring sites have been considered (Nishi, 1993).

Biochemical effect of vascular bubbles

In vitro studies have shown that gas bubbles affect cells and disrupt biochemical processes. Thorsen could show that gas bubbles are associated with aggregation of thrombocytes; the degree of aggregation being independent of the gas content of the bubble but is rather related its surface properties (Thorsen et al., 1986). Independently, Ward and Bergh have reported that gas bubbles activate complement in-vitro and the response is unrelated to the

TABLE 1. DOPPLER GRADES (PRECORDIAL) IN DIFFERENT STUDIES AND DCI INCIDENCE

AUTHORS		NO BUBBLES	GRADES I-IV
Spencer and Johanson, 1974	n	110	64
	% DCI	1.0	22
Gotoh and Nashimoto, 1977	n	64	88
	% DCI	0	19
Marroni and Zannini, 1981	n	64	33
	% DCI	0	9
Nishi, 1993	n	1265	331
	% DCI	0.6	8
Brubakk et al., 1991	n	68	40
	% DCI	1.5	7.5

Modified from Brubakk, 2003

content of the bubble. This also supports the hypothesis that the bioactive properties of bubbles are related to their surface characteristics (Ward, 1967; Bergh et al., 1993). Ward also differentiated between "sensitive" and "non-sensitive" individuals, depending on the degree of complement activation in response to bubbles. The latter has also been related to clinical manifestations of DCI. Individuals with low C5a levels before dives produced many gas bubbles. A single air dive also reduced C5a levels suggesting that gas bubbles may activate both C5a and C5a receptors. Stevens has confirmed this phenomenon in divers for up to 14 hours after being treated for DCI (Stevens et al., 1993).

Complement activation triggers the activation of neutrophils and the formation of multiple membrane attack complexes (MAC) that eventually lead to cellular destruction (Kilgore et al., 1994). This also causes the leukocytes to adhere to the endothelium as they circulate over damaged endothelium. Such neutrophil activation has been demonstrated during decompression (Benestad et al., 1990).

Some of the skin changes seen in DCI may be related to C5a activation: erythema, edema and infiltration of inflammatory cells (Swerlick et al., 1988). Other important effects of C5a are vasoconstriction and blood flow reduction (Martin et al., 1988).

Interestingly, post ischemic increases in blood flow (i.e., hyperemia) are not seen—possibly due the prolonged effects related to C5a activation, leukocyte adherence or even persisting vascular or perivascular bubbles (Bergh et al., 1993). If circulation of blood becomes restricted during decompression, gas elimination would be similarly reduced possibly leading to critical supersaturation and local bubble formation.

Vik, et al. have also observed that pulmonary changes in pigs following decompression were similar to those observed after complement activation. Lungs exposed to significant amounts of bubbles for approximately 100 minutes after decompression developed considerable leukocyte invasion (Vik et al., 1990). Complement activation was therefore considered to be the most important mechanism for acute lung injury (Ward, 1967; Ward et al., 1995).

Certain pulmonary function changes have been observed in divers. These include a reduction in carbon monoxide diffusion capacity and compliance (Thorsen et al., 1986). They are believed to support the growing evidence that inflammatory processes may follow decompression. In fact the reduction in carbon monoxide diffusion capacity is rapid and is associated with the development of bubbles (Dujic et al., 1992; Dujic et al., 1993).

Brubakk, et al. consider the lungs to be a primary target organ for gas bubbles. It is probably exposed to gas bubble effects following all decompressions. Indeed the concept of the lungs serving as a "bubble trap" has been purported for many years, but we are only now starting to look at the impact this function has on the "filter" itself.

Although removal of bubbles by the lungs prevents more harmful distribution of bubbles to the arterial system, the filtering mechanism is not foolproof. If the gas load on the lungs is large, the filtering capabilities of the lungs will eventually be exceeded and gas will enter the arterial circulation. An increase in pulmonary artery pressure of only about 30% is considered sufficient to cause arterialization of venous gas bubbles (Vik et al., 1990).

Central nervous system changes in DCI are believed to result from multiple mechanisms, including intra- and extravascular (tissue) bubbles (Francis et al., 1990).

Vascular bubbles no longer seem to be the primary pathophysiological feature of short latency, acute spinal cord DCI. In a group of ten amateur and ten professional divers, five of whom had neurological DCI, no vascular changes could be seen (Morild and Mork, 1994).

However the same authors reported changes in the endothelial layer of the brain ventricles in a group of divers (Morild and Mork, 1994; Mork et al., 1994).

Brubakk has entertained the possibility that this may not so much be evidence of intravascular gas bubbles as it may be indicative of an increase in venous pressure due to venous gas embolism of the lung interfering with venous return. Another possible explanation may be gas bubbles in the spinal fluid adhering to the lining of the ventricles and causing changes in the adjacent endothelium (Brubakk, 1994). Indeed, Chryssantou has shown that animals exposed to decompression show changes in the integrity of the blood-brain-barrier, while Broman has confirmed that even short contact between gas bubbles and endothelium (i.e., 1–2 minutes) leads to such changes (Broman et al., 1966; Chryssanthou et al., 1977). Further studies in rabbits have shown that bubble-endothelium contact causes endothelial damage and a progressive reduction in cerebral blood flow and function (Helps and Gorman, 1991).

CLINICAL MANIFESTATIONS OF DCI

There is an ongoing controversy about the best way to classify dysbaric illnesses. Until 1990, these disorders were divided into DCS and AGE. DCS was then divided into two broad categories based on the severity of symptoms and the associated treatment regimens. However, today we recognize that certain forms of DCS may be the result of paradoxical or even frank AGE; therefore, in the application of the traditional classification that follows, a modifier (i.e., either DCS or DCI) is added to indicate where such pathophysiological ambiguity exists.[†]

Mild (Previously called 'Type I'):
- Limb pain ("bends")—DCS
- Lymphatic manifestations—DCS
- Cutaneous manifestations—DCI

Serious (previously called 'Type II'):
- Pulmonary manifestations—DCI (or "chokes")
- Central Nervous System (brain, spinal cord and peripheral nerves) and Audiovestibular (Inner Ear) manifestations—DCI
- Shock—DCI
- Abdominal, Thoracic or Back Pain—DCI
- Extreme fatigue, constitutional symptoms or general malaise—DCI

---

† Certain manifestations of decompression disorders are known never to be associated with gas embolism and therefore can confidently be classified as decompression sickness. These include limb "bends" and lymphatic DCS.

Time to Onset of Symptoms (all manifestions)
- 50% occur within 30 minutes of surfacing
- 85% occur within 1 hour of surfacing
- 95% occur within 3 hours of surfacing
- 1% delayed more than 12 hours

However, initial symptoms have been reported more than 24 hours after surfacing particularly if there is subsequent altitude exposure (e.g., flying or mountaineering).

Mild form:

Pain—DCS

In recreational compressed air diving, the upper extremities are involved three times more frequently than the lower limbs. This is reversed for caisson workers and in commercial saturation diving. The pain can range from slight discomfort to a dull, deep, boring or even unbearable pain. It is usually unaffected by movement of the joint and there may be overlying edema and regional numbness.

Lymphatic manifestations—DCS

Lymphatic DCS is presumably the consequence of obstruction of lymphatics by bubbles. The manifestations can include pain and swelling of lymph nodes, with lymphedema of the tissues drained by the obstructed lymph nodes. New data are suggesting that normobaric oxygen may improve the flow of lymph and may assist in resolving inert gas bubbles contained within the lymphatic system (Balestra et al., 2004a).

Cutaneous manifestations—DCI

Cutaneous forms of decompression illness fall into two broad categories, superficial (diver's lice / erythema) and deep vascular (cutis marmorata).

- *Diver's Lice / Erythema*: Itching is common following decompression from dry chamber dives where the skin is in direct contact with the chamber atmosphere rather than in water. This condition—sometimes called "diver's lice"—is thought to be the result of gas dissolving directly into the skin and causing cutaneous irritation and the release of histamine with itchiness upon decompression. This is not a true or systemic form of DCI and does not require recompression. On the other hand, itchiness or redness of the skin following a dive in which the skin was wet, is more likely to be true cutaneous DCI.[†] However, this is usually accompanied by some degree of skin rash or visible skin change.
- *Cutis Marmorata*: This form of DCI is thought to result from a complex interaction between bubbles, venous congestion and the immune system. It usually manifests as bluish-red "blotches"—frequently affecting the upper back and chest. Prominent linear purple markings are also frequently observed. These manifestations are a systemic form of

---

† Note that some in-water dives are performed in drysuits. Under these conditions the skin is also in direct contact with compressed gas and "divers lice" may appear.

DCI; they suggest significant bubble formation, which may also be affecting other areas of the body. Prompt recompression is usually recommended and typically leads to prompt resolution. This sign may be a herald of more serious forms of DCI and there is an association with PFO that will be discussed later.

Serious form:

Pulmonary—DCI[†]

Pulmonary DCI usually presents as a triad of symptoms:

- Substernal pain—usually burning and progressively increasing. Initially the pain may be noted only when coughing or with deep inspiration. Over time, the pain may become constant.
- Cough—initially intermittent and provoked by cigarette smoking (Behnke's sign). Paroxysms of coughing may become intractable.
- Progressive respiratory distress (dyspnea).

The manifestations of pulmonary DCI are related to the combined effects of gas emboli in the pulmonary artery and obstruction of the vascular supply to the bronchial mucosa. Untreated pulmonary DCI may be fatal.

Neurological—DCI

Although the exact mechanism of neurological DCI is not fully understood it is believed to include embolism, autochthonous (i.e., spontaneous extravascular/interstitial bubble formation), venous stasis and immunological phenomena. These mechanisms have different latencies and show different responses to recompression. The neurological manifestations of DCI are therefore unpredictable and any abnormalities in relation to diving are subject to suspicion: *Any neurological abnormality following a dive should be assumed the result of neurological DCI until proven otherwise.*

Cerebral—DCI

Brain involvement in DCI appears to be especially common in high-altitude aviators (i.e., flying in excess of 25,000 feet in unpressurized aircraft). In this group, pulmonary venous gas embolism is also common and hypoxia and positive pressure breathing may facilitate the transfer of bubbles or immunological products into the systemic circulation. Not surprisingly, a migraine-like headache accompanied by visual disturbances, is a common manifestation of high-altitude DCI. In divers, brain involvement usually presents more overtly with stroke-like symptoms.

Collapse with unconsciousness is a rare presentation of DCI but common in AGE. If it does occur, it represents a very serious form of DCI.

Spinal cord—DCI

Paraplegia is a "classic" manifestation of DCI in divers and represents spinal cord involvement. Bladder paralysis with urinary retention and fecal incontinence frequently accompany such paraplegia.

---

† Not pulmonary barotrauma or AGE.

Recent years have seen a decline in both the proportion and absolute number of cases of serious paralysis in recreational divers: from 13.4% in 1987 to only 2.9% in 1997. Similarly loss of consciousness has dropped from 7.4% to 3.9% during the same period; the incidence of loss of bladder function has dropped from 2.2% to 0.4% during this period (DAN Diving Accident Reports).

Interestingly, the reduction in severe neurological symptoms has not been balanced by a proportional rise in pain-only or skin manifestations. Rather there has been an unexpected appearance of mild, ambiguous neurological manifestations, such as paresthesia or tingling, which nevertheless appear to respond well to oxygen administration and recompression.

Inner ear—DCI

Audiovestibular DCI is a relatively rare manifestation of CNS involvement. Frequently, though not always, both the cochlea and vestibular apparatus are involved so that the presenting signs and symptoms may include tinnitus, deafness, vertigo, nausea, vomiting and ataxia. Nystagmus may be present on physical examination.

The exact mechanism is not clear. Bubble formation in perilymph and embolization of the auditory/vestibular artery are plausible possibilities (Cantais et al., 2003).

Inner ear DCI is a serious medical emergency and must be treated immediately to avoid permanent damage. Since the nutrient arteries of the inner ear are very small, rapid reduction in bubble diameter, with immediate 100% oxygen administration and prompt recompression, are essential.

Shock—DCI

Shock is a rare manifestation of DCI. It is often associated with serious pulmonary problems and may be life threatening. Multiple mechanisms may contribute to the development of shock. These include: loss of vascular tone due to spinal cord involvement; myocardial depression due to accumulation of venous gas bubbles in the cardiac chambers with air-locking; hypoxemia and acidosis; pulmonary embolization; and hypovolemia due to increased capillary leakage with loss of intravascular volume and blood thickening (hemoconcentration).

Back, abdominal, or chest pain—DCI

Unlike simple limb or joint pain, constricting back, abdominal or chest pain may indicate spinal cord involvement and should be examined carefully.

Extreme fatigue—DCI

Disproportionate or extreme tiredness after diving, which cannot be explained by preceding physical exertion, is associated with serious DCI. It may be due to the release of biochemical mediators in response to the entrapment of venous gas emboli in pulmonary vascular beds. As such, the condition may deteriorate with the appearance of serious pulmonary symptoms or a variety of neurological manifestations.

NEW DCI CLASSIFICATION

The simple classification of Type I and II DCS suggests that the different categories of decompression sickness fall within clearly defined clinical boundaries. This being the case, there should be reasonable concordance in the application of this classification system (Brubakk, 1994; Brubakk and Eftedal, 2001). However, Smith and Kemper—in two separate studies—have shown considerable disparity between experts applying this classification system to the same cases. For instance, several cases of cerebral DCI could not be clearly distinguished from arterial gas embolism or inner ear barotrauma.[†]

Other studies have shown that musculoskeletal manifestations are regularly accompanied by neurological symptoms (Vann et al., 1993; Freiberger et al., 2002). This confirms that DCS manifestations may fall within both categories; Type I and II are therefore non-exclusive. Perhaps more importantly, in the

TABLE 2. CLASSIFICATION OF SYMPTOMS IN DCI

		Definitions>	ABRUPT	EVOLVING	STATIC
		Onset Time>	IMMEDIATE	FIRST DAY	DAYS TO YEARS
LOCALIZATION	SOMATIC	PAINFUL	Limb Bend Periarticular pain	Limb Bend: fluctuating pain after dive	Osteonecrosis
		PARESTHETIC	Tingling or numbness, may herald spinal DCI	Tingling or numbness, may be combined with pain	Recurrent or episodic after treatment; probably benign
		ASYMPTOMATIC	Skin changes or painless swelling	Skin changes or painless swelling	Asymptomatic Osteonecrosis
	CEREBRAL		Loss of consciousness, hemiplegia, "air embolism"	Hemiparesis, delirium, brainstem signs, vertigo	Chronic neuropsycho-logical changes
	SPINAL		Girdle pain, loss of leg movement and bladder control	Waxing and waning, weakness, bladder dys-function, sensory levels	Chronic gait and bladder disturbances
	CEREBRO-SPINAL		Unconscious diver with spinal findings	Combined spinal and cerebral signs, varying	Combined cerebral and spinal disability; spinal predominates
	SYSTEMIC		Chokes; acute systemic respiratory collapse	Fatigue, rare visceral DCI	Rare cases of ARDS and lung damage

absence of careful examination, the more serious manifestations could be overlooked and the cases could be erroneously assigned to Type I DCS. For example, extreme fatigue could either be classified as a minor symptom or a sign of subclinical pulmonary embolism (Hallenbeck et al., 1975).

As a result of all these deficiencies, Francis, et al. proposed the now wide-ly accepted term "DCI" and its associated classification system (Francis and Smith, 1991). The latter encompasses both categories of decompression sick-ness and arterial gas embolism.

---

† Note that biphasic DCI - previously called 'Type 3 DCS' is not considered in the text. The condition refers to AGE from pulmonary barotrauma evolving into neurological DCS.

Importantly, instead of being a categorical system, it is a descriptive one based on clinical manifestations (signs and/or symptoms) and their evolution over time. Using this classification scheme, a very high degree of concordance could be achieved between different specialists (Pollard et al., 1995). Francis and Smith have also proposed the following Classification Table for DCI. This offers a useful guide to correctly describe the various possible manifestations of dysbaric disorders / DCI (Francis and Smith, 1991).

TREATMENT OF DCI[†]

Air was used universally as a breathing gas during recompression for the first half of the 20th century. Oxygen recompression treatment was not really considered until Yarbrough and Behnke's preliminary experiments in 1939 (Yarbrough and Behnke, 1939). In fact it was only after the work of Workman and Goodman that this became standard practice (Workman, 1965).

Early treatment approaches were essentially homeopathic in that they were recreating the conditions under which the disease had occurred. The challenge was deciding how much recompression was required and how long the process of decompression should last. The original depth of the dive was used as a guide. For example, if a 40-meter dive led to symptoms, recompression to the same pressure would be expected to alleviate them. However, there was controversy about whether the depth of relief of clinical symptoms or the depth of the dive was most important. Ultimately, a compromise was reached by recommending depth of relief plus one atmosphere. The rationale was that if a bubble became small enough, surface tension would cause it to collapse and disappear. It was clearly understood that any bubbles remaining in the tissues and circulation would continue to take up inert gas as more nitrogen was absorbed during the recompression treatment.

In the 1924 edition of the U.S. Navy Diving Manual, a series of air recompression tables were introduced. Unfortunately, more than 50% of treatments were unsuccessful. In 1945, Van Der Aue and Behnke experimented with better treatment methods. This led to the publication of the U.S. Navy air recompression tables I to IV that became the world standard for the next 20 years. Outcomes improved to nearly 90% recovery rates (Van Der Aue et al., 1945). In spite of their 10% failure rate and somewhat daunting durations (6h 20 for Table I; 38h 11 for Table IV), these tables were considered very successful and represented the best therapeutic solutions available at the time.

By 1963, however, the observed failure rate of serious symptoms approached 46% on initial recompression and this rose to 47.1% in 1964. The failure was attributed to a greater number of treated civilians. Many of these had dived in total ignorance of decompression schedules, not to mention the fact that their delay to treatment was significantly longer than for most military divers. Consequently, Goodman and Workman started investigating the use of oxygen at moderate depths (2.8 ATA) for the treatment of DCI (Workman, 1965). Oxygen treatment had first been suggested by Behnke in 1939. At that time, however, the U.S. Navy Bureau of Medicine and Surgery was concerned that oxygen breathing in the chamber may be dangerous and not "sailor

---

† Treatment of deep or satiation diving falls outside the scope or this section. It refers to conventional recreational diving only.

proof" and that the risks of oxygen toxicity and fire were too great (Kindwall, 1998). For this reason, Behnke's excellent results were ignored. Ironically, Edgar End in Milwaukee had already introduced oxygen breathing in 1947 with excellent results in over 250 cases of DCI in compressed air workers (Kindwall, 1998).

The first 52 cases treated with the "new" Goodman and Workman oxygen schemes showed that 30 minutes at the maximum depth of 18 meters and total oxygen breathing treatment time of 90 minutes could be considered minimum or "adequate" treatment, allowing for a 3.6% failure rate. Oxygen breathing schedules were lengthened to two hours for mild and four hours for serious symptoms, with intermittent air breathing intervals of 5 to 15 minutes to avoid oxygen toxicity. The two and four hour schemes were called U.S. Navy Table 5 and 6 respectively and were officially published in 1967. The most significant conceptual difference from the previous approach, was the importance given to the time of relief, rather than the depth of relief (Kindwall, 1998). Now that a gas other than nitrogen was being used, it was no longer necessary to keep the bubble small under pressure until they collapsed on their own. Nitrogen could actively be eliminated by oxygen whereas pressure now simply became the vehicle whereby this drug—oxygen —could be introduced to correct the underlying damage. This approach therefore offered a dual benefit.

Now that oxygen treatments had been established as the standard of care, the next major controversy was whether to offer prolonged or repetitive treatments. Although serial treatments of DCI were already advocated by many, consensus was only reached in 1976 at a meeting of the North Sea off-shore diving groups at the Royal Society of Medicine in London. It was agreed that if the diver had residual symptoms after the initial treatment, daily oxygen recompression should be continued for at least two weeks or until the patient's signs and symptoms had plateaued (Elliott et al., 1974a, 1974b; Elliott and Moon, 1993; Eke et al., 2000).

By the late 60's and 70's, adjunctive pharmacological treatment was introduced to complement recompression therapy. In 1979, the Undersea Medical Society organized a workshop on the management of severe and complicated cases of DCI, where the importance of hydration, steroids, heparin, aspirin and other agents were discussed.

Although, the US Navy Table 6 remains the most commonly used recompression schedule to this day, various modifications and alternatives have been introduced over the years. The Comex 30 Table, using mixed gas at a maximum pressure of four atmospheres, has its proponents, while saturation treatments (e.g., USN TT7) have also started featuring more recently. First introduced by Miller in 1978, saturation treatment typically started at four atmospheres with the patient breathing oxygen at 0.35 to 0.5 ATA (Miller et al., 1978). Nevertheless, in spite of the availability of a number of alternatives, the available evidence still supports the use of USN TT6 for most DCI cases where treatment can be initiated promptly (DAN Diving Accident Reports).

Unfortunately, there are often very considerable delays in initiating treatment, and many of the secondary effects of the bubbles on blood and tissues then become important. Kelleher has shown that initial treatment is effective in only about 66% of such cases (Kelleher et al., 1996). However, by this time the failure is probably no longer due to deficiencies in the recompression schedule but rather because the delays have made the injuries permanent. Alternative protocols, including saturation decompression, have not proven to be superior to US Navy Table 6 (Leitch and Barnard, 1982; Leitch, 1985). The use of different gas mixes—particularly heliox—while showing promise (Hyldegaard and Madsen, 1989; Hyldegaard et al., 1991; Hyldegaard and Madsen, 1994), still remain controversial in the treatment of DCI from air diving.

The severity of symptoms and delay are not the only considerations in outcome and treatment effectiveness. Heliox and Trimix dives may differ from air dives due to the differences in partition coefficients of helium and nitrogen in the tissues (Brubakk et al., 1986).

With access to recompression being an important limiting factor, various efforts have been made to replace or improve the treatment of DCI with certain drugs, generally with little success. Some of these show promise in experimental work. Lutz and Herrmann have been able to substantially reduce the mortality of rats undergoing rapid decompression from 8 ATA when fluorocarbons were infused after decompression (Lutz and Herrmann, 1984). Drugs, such as lidocaine, may also have a role in attenuating leukocyte-endothelium adhesion related to complement activation (Evans et al., 1988; Mitchell, 2001).

In 1994, the European Committee for Hyperbaric Medicine organized its first European Consensus Conference. DCI was one of the topics. In 1996 a second, more specific Consensus Conference was organized. The theme of the conference was "The Treatment of Decompression Accidents in Recreational Diving." Following both Conferences and extensive presentations by leading international experts, two International Juries formulated recommendations that have since been adopted in Europe as the current standard for the treatment of DCI. These are summarized in the following section.

CONCLUSION

DCI is generally considered a relatively benign condition: If adequate treatment is started promptly, complete clinical resolution may be achieved in 80–90% of cases. There is universal consensus that 100% oxygen should be administered immediately. It is the single most important first aid treatment in any DCI case associated with surface-oriented diving. In addition, rehydration is a very valuable adjunct during field first aid management of such cases.

Hyperbaric treatment should be started promptly upon the appearance of DCI manifestations. Hyperbaric treatment tables using 100% oxygen at environmental pressures not exceeding 2.8 ATA, with various depth/time modifications, show consistently good results in more than 80% of the treated cases. There is no significant evidence suggesting that better alternatives exist. Accordingly, USN TT6 or its equivalent remains the first choice for the treatment of DCI related to surface-oriented diving.

Many specialists agree that the use of high pressure (generally 4 ATA maximum) treatment tables using a gas mixture of 50% Helium and 50% Oxygen may prove highly effective and provide good results in the cases that do not respond quickly and satisfactorily to the standard low pressure hyperbaric oxygen treatment tables.

Although conclusive scientific evidence on pharmacological treatment is limited, the administration of adjunctive fluid therapy is considered very important and generally recommended by diving and hyperbaric medicine specialists. The role of other drugs, such as steroids and anticoagulants, although widely used without any apparent adverse effect, remains controversial.

In cases where the initial DCI treatment tables achieve complete resolution, residual neurological problems should be managed by providing follow-up recompression as well as specific rehabilitation.

CHAPTER 2

OTHER ADVERSE EFFECTS OF SCUBA DIVING

INTRODUCTION

The history of modern diving dates back to the development of the first self-contained underwater breathing apparatus (SCUBA) by Charles Condert in 1831. Although military diving developed steadily, the rise of recreational scuba diving only occurred after 1943 when Emile Gagnan and Jacques-Yves Cousteau invented an automatic SCUBA demand valve.

Today, recreational or sport diving has become very popular. There are more than 4 million scuba divers in the North America; more than 1 million in Europe; 250,000 in southern Africa; 500,000 in Australia and New Zealand; and 150,000 in Japan. An additional 200,000 new scuba divers are trained internationally every year and many millions of recreational dives are performed annually. The ignorant still consider SCUBA diving a "high risk" sport even though statistics clearly show otherwise; it is a most forgiving sport.

PROFESSIONAL/COMMERCIAL VERSUS RECREATIONAL/SPORT SCUBA DIVING BEHAVIOR

Professional and sport diving have much in common; both use underwater breathing apparatus and similar supportive gear. The scope of professional diving, however, is much wider than sport diving. Commercial and other interests impose greater depths, longer durations and more challenging diving conditions on commercial divers. For the diving professional, the task dictates the method and nature of their dive. For sport divers, on the other hand, enjoyment, simplicity and safety usually define their diving practices. These differences obviously affect the nature and number of injuries and fatalities between the groups.

Ironically, in many respects, professional divers carry out their activities in a much more regulated and controlled environment than sport divers do. Accidents are also more likely to be reported and, when they do occur, treatment is usually at hand so that the long-term effects are frequently less severe. Dives usually involve better planning, more adherence to the dive plan, and more extensive surface support.

DCI, FATALITIES AND OTHER ACCIDENTS—INCIDENCE IN PROFESSIONAL VERSUS SPORT SCUBA DIVERS

The dependence on a breathable gas source; the need for consciousness to maintain an intact airway; and the requirement of some physical capability to ensure self-preservation while in water, make diving a potentially hazardous sport (Hardy, 1997). Yet diving fatalities are usually associated with panic (Morgan, 1995)—an avoidable problem—while diving injuries and accidents are usually minor in nature and commonly the result of ear and sinus barotraumas. Other injuries may include near-drowning and DCI. Nevertheless, as pointed out by Bennett and Elliott, we have no accurate figures for scuba diving accidents (Bennett and Elliott, 1993).

There has also been an ongoing concern that the reported incidence of DCI in professional divers is artificially low. Upon the introduction of anonymous reporting, there was a 25% increase in cases; it appeared that one or more individuals in the workforce is being injured on 42.5% of working days (Kindwall, 1998). As for the Navy, Murrison et al. suggested in 1991 that there seemed to be an increasing trend in diving accidents over a ten-year study period. They reported an average of 1.9 accidents per 1000 dive hours; one accident per 88 divers; and 2.3 fatalities per 10,000 divers (Murrison et al., 1991).

In the US military community on Okinawa Island, Arness performed a retrospective study of diving accidents over a seven-year period. He reported an average of 13.4 annual DCI events per 100,000 dives with a fatality incidence of 1.3 per 100.000 dives (Arness, 1997).

Divers Alert Network (DAN) presently offers the best information on recreational scuba diving injuries and fatalities. Based on the estimated number of SCUBA participants the DCI incidence has been estimated between one case of DCI for every 1,700 to 4,000 divers per year (Di Tullio et al., 1993a). In addition, in a four-year retrospective study, they reported two fatalities per 100,000 divers. This is one order of magnitude lower than the figure for professional scuba divers.

Based on accident reports, DAN has noticed that the number of fatalities has decreased from 8.62 per 100,000 dives in 1976 to 2.74–3.2 per 100,000 dives in 1992—an encouraging sign.

Finally, it should be noted that the US national safety council (an organization collecting and reporting on accidents in general) reported in 1991 that the accident rate for scuba diving was considered very low (i.e., 0.04%) similar to bowls. By way of comparison, the accident rates for some other sports are as follows: tennis (0.12%), football (0.91%), baseball (2.09%) and American football (2.17%).

Given that most diving injuries are related to ear or sinus barotraumas (Marroni 1991), the overall risk of decompression-related injuries in the global recreational diving population is very low. As further confirmation of the relative safety of underwater diving as a sport, and the positive impact of proper training, this combined data analysis from the University of Rhode Island and PADI International shows that whilst the number of diving trainees is clearly on the increase, the number of fatalities is not.

TABLE 1. OCCURRENCE OF INJURIES IN VARIOUS SPORTS

Sport	Participants	Injuries	Incidence
Football	14,700,000	319,157	2.17%
Baseball	15,400,000	321,806	2.09%
Basketball	26,200,000	486,920	1.86%
Soccer	11,200,000	101,946	0.91%
Volleyball	25,100,000	92,961	0.37%
Water Skiing	10,800,000	21,499	0.20%
Racquetball	8,200,000	13,795	0.17%
Tennis	18,800,000	22,507	0.12%
Swimming	70,500,000	65,757	0.09%
Bowling	40,800,000	17,351	0.04%
SCUBA Diving	**2,600,000**	**1,044**	**0.04%**

From Accident Facts, 1991—National Safety Council, USA; National Sporting Goods Association, USA; and National Electronic Injury Survey System (NEISS), USA. Numbers represent individuals who participate in the sport more than once per year; injury represents someone who was treated in an emergency room for an accident relating to the sport or involving sport equipment.

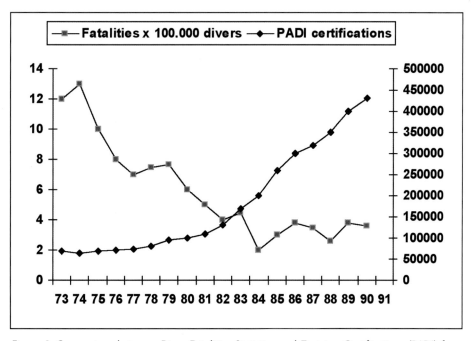

Figure 1. Comparison between Diver Fatalities Statistics and Training Certifications (PADI) from 1973 until 1990.

NOTES

SECTION 2
PATENCY OF FORAMEN OVALE AND SCUBA DIVING

CHAPTER 3

DEVELOPMENT OF THE FETAL HEART

DEVELOPMENT OF THE ATRIA

To understand the adult anatomy of the atria, their embryological development needs to be considered. This is important because it explains the possible abnormal development of various intracardiac structures, and it provides the terminology with which to describe them in both the fetal and adult heart. The descriptions are based on the works of Testut and Latarjet (Testut and Latarjet, 1948; Patten, 1953; Moore and Bignold, 1988; Sadler, 1990a).

During embryogenesis, the heart evolves from a tube with a continuous blood flow to a complex four-chambered organ with pulsatile flow. During this morphogenesis, the circulation is partitioned in a right-sided pulmonary and left-sided systemic circulation without an interruption in the continuous flow. The pulmonary circulation remains immature until after birth, when breathing commences. Following birth, both the pulmonary and systemic circulations receive equal amounts of blood.

Primordial Tubular Heart

The heart appears in the middle of the third week. It arises from paired primordia situated ventrolaterally beneath the pharynx, in-between the prochordal and neural plate (Figure 1). After closure of the neural plate and the formation of the brain vesicle, the central nervous system grows so rapidly in a cephalic direction that it extends over the central cardiogenic area and the future pericardial cavity. With this, the prochordal plate, the later buccopharyngeal membrane, and the central portion of the cardiogenic plate are pulled forward, and rotate over 180 degrees along a transverse axis. The central part of the cardiogenic plate and pericardial cavity move ventrally and caudally toward the buccopharyngeal membrane (Figure 1). Simultaneously, the initially flat embryo folds in the transverse dimension, resulting in the approximation of the two lateral endocardial tubes and fusion from cranial to caudal (Figure 2). This primitive endocardial tube bulges progressively into the pericardial cavity and is attached with a dorsal double-layered supporting membrane, the *mesocardium dorsale*. In this manner, the nearly straight double wall tube is suspended medially, for a time, in the anterior part of the coelom. The surrounding mesoderm, adjacent to the endocardial tube, condenses at the same time, forming the epimyocardial mantle. The cardiac jelly separates the two layers, which are invaded progressively by endothelium. Finally, the

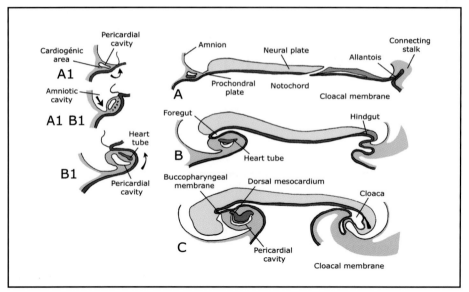

Figure 1. The heart tube growing during early embryonic life. Schematic longitudinal sections through the embryos at different stages of development show the formation of the pericardial cavity from primordial A, 17 days; B, 18 days; C, 22 days (Sadler, 1990b; Sadler and Langman, 2000, 2004).

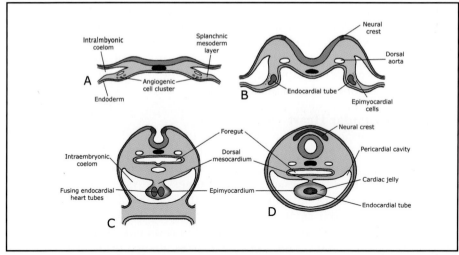

Figure 2. Embryo schematic transverse sections. Schematic transverse section through the embryos at different stages of development showing the formation of a single heart tube from paired primordial A, 17 days; B, 18 days; C, 21 days; D, 22 days (after (Sadler, 1990b; Sadler and Langman, 2000, 2004).

tube is formed by three layers: 1) the *endocardium*—destined to become the internal lining of the heart; 2) the *myocardium*—the muscular layer of the heart wall, formed by the migration of a myoepicardium mantle from the inner aspect of the visceral pericardium; and finally 3) the *epicardium*—derived from the *lamina visceralis*, covering the outside of the tube. The tube has at its cephalic side the arterial pole with efferent vessels of the embryo, and at its caudal side the venous pole with the afferent vessels.

Figure 1 is made up of a series of schematic drawings showing the result of the rapid growth of the brain vesicles on the position of the pericardial cavity and the process of growth of the developing heart tube. Initially, the cardiogenic area and pericardial cavity are located in front of the prochordal plate. Because of the rotation along a transverse axis through the prochordal plate, the cardiogenic area (heart tube) finally comes to lie dorsally to the pericardial cavity. This is most apparent in the embryo between 18 and 22 days (Sadler, 1990b; Sadler and Langman, 2000, 2004).

THE CARDIAC LOOP AND THE ESTABLISHMENT OF REGIONAL DIVISION OF THE HEART

The segment enveloped in the pericardial cavity is originally straight. The intra-pericardial part consists of the future bulboventricular portion, whereas the atrial portion and sinus venosus lie outside the *pericardium* as paired structures (Figure 3A). Due to rapid elongation of the cardiac tube, regional differentiation occurs with a series of constrictions along its length with bending. As both ends of the tube are anchored—the cephalic end to the aortic roots and the caudal end to the great veins—the intermediate portion undergoes the greatest change in shape (Figure 3B). This process is accompanied by the breakdown of the dorsal mesocardium. The cephalic portion of the tube extends in a ventral and caudal direction towards the right, while the caudal atrial portion shifts in a dorsocranial direction to the left, creating the cardiac loop (Figure 3C). The sinus venosus, initially a paired structure, enters the pericardial cavity (Figures 3C and 4A). The atrial region is established by transverse dilatation of the tubular heart, cephalic of the sinus venosus. The atrioventricular junction remains narrow and forms the atrioventricular canal. The *bulbus cordis*, in its proximal portion, forms the trabeculated part of the right ventricle; in its mid portion (i.e., the *conus cordis*) it forms the outflow tract of both ventricles; and in its distal portion (i.e., *trun-*

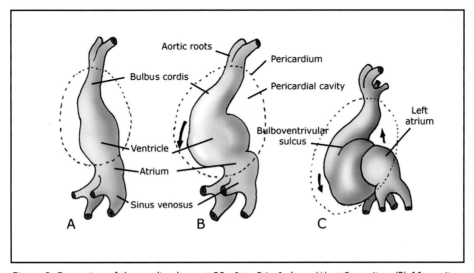

Figure 3. Formation of the cardiac loop at 23±1 to 24±1 days. (A) at 8 somites; (B) 11 somites; and (C) 16 somites (from Sadler, 1990b; Sadler and Langman, 2000, 2004).

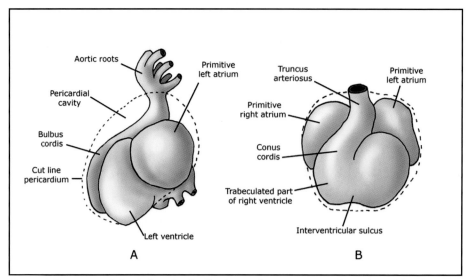

Figure 4. Formation of the *Bulbus Cordis*. The heart of an approximately 28 days old embryo. (A) as seen from the left; (B) as seen from the front. The partitioning of the truncus and conus and the formation of the membranous portion of the interventricular septum. The bulbus cordis is divided into the truncus arteriosus, the conus cordis, and the trabecular part of right ventricle (Sadler, 1990b; Sadler and Langman, 2000, 2004).

cus arteriosus) it forms the aorta and pulmonary artery roots (Figure 4B). The further development of this single streamed tube into a dual circulation follows division of the tube.

DEVELOPMENT OF THE SINUS VENOSUS

The *sinus venosus* develops as a paired structure in the middle of the fourth week. It is made up of a central transverse portion and two extensions: the right and left sinus horn (Figure 5A). The sinus drains the vitelline, the umbilical, and the common cardinal veins to the atrial primordium, generally recognized as the primitive atrium. At first, the communication is wide, but soon the entrance of the sinus shifts to the right during the fourth and fifth weeks of development. As a result, there is successive obliteration of the left umbilical vein, the left vitelline vein, and finally the left common cardinal vein, following which the importance of the left sinus horn decreases. The oblique vein of the left atrium and the coronary sinus are the only structures that drain into the left sinus horn (Figure 5B). In contrast, the right horn enlarges and forms the only communication between the sinus venosus and the atrium. The complete junction invaginates itself into the primitive atrium as a bilaminated funnel and forms the right and left venous valves of the sinuatrial orifice (Figure 6). The valves fuse dorsocranially, forming a ridge known as the *septum spurium*. Finally, the right horn is incorporated into the right atrium to form the smooth walled atrial part (Figure 5B). The left venous valve and the *septum spurium* fuse with the developing atrial septum. The superior portion of the right sinus valve disappears, and the inferior portion develops into the valve of the inferior vena cava (Eustachius) and the valve of the coronary sinus (Thebesius) (Figure 5C). The crista terminalis is the dividing line

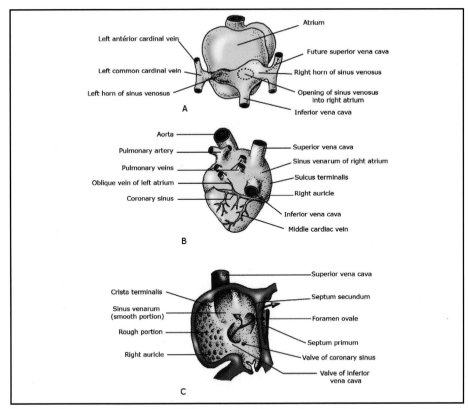

Figure 5. *Sinus venosus* formation. (A) Dorsal view of the heart at about 26 days shows the *sinus venosus*; the umbilical and vitilline veins are not shown; (B) Dorsal view at eight weeks after incorporation of the right horn of the sinus venosus into the right atrium. The left horn of the sinus venosus has become the coronary sinus. (C) Internal view of the fetal right atrium showing 1) the smooth part of the wall of the right atrium (sinus venarum) derived from the right horn of the sinus venosus and 2) the crista terminalis and the valves of the inferior vena cava and coronary sinus derived from the right sinoatrial valve. The primitive right atrium becomes the right auricle, a conical muscular pouch, which lies against the root of the aorta in the adult (Moore 1988).

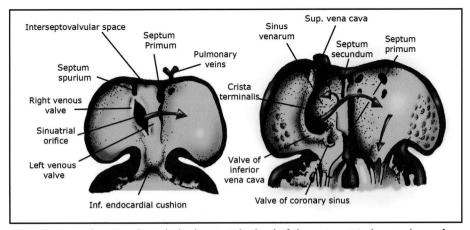

Figure 6. Coronal section through the heart at the level of the atrioventricular canal seen from the ventral view to show the development of the sinus valves at a 7–8 mm stage (Sadler, 1990b; Sadler and Langman, 2000, 2004).

between the original atrium, formed by the trabeculated atrial appendage containing the pectinate muscles, and the smooth-walled part originating from the right sinus horn, forming the *sinus venarum* (Figure 5C).

SEPTATION OF THE ATRIA

Atrial septation requires the delivery of right systemic venous blood to the right side of the atrium, with the concurrent development of pulmonary circulation. The latter develops in the lung buds, situated at the posterior side of the heart as outgrowths of the foregut. Initially, the intrapulmonary venous plexus is connected to the splanchnic venous plexus rather than the venous pole of the heart tube.

During embryonic development, there is a dramatic reorganization of blood flow in the venous channels. Through the development of anastomic channels, most of the left-sided blood (i.e., blood normally streaming to the left sinus horn), is diverted towards the right sided veins. The end-result is the obliteration of veins draining into the left sinus horn, with the exception of the oblique vein of the left atrium and the coronary sinus. At the end of organogenesis, the right vitelline and the right cardinal veins are the only remaining channels toward the sinus venosus. With the shift of the sinuatrial junction and the decrease in size of the left sinus horn, the sinuatrial junction now opens to the right side of the primitive atrium. Simultaneously, a primary pulmonary vein grows at the posterior side of the left atrium, between the enlarged sinus horn, and the regressing left sinus horn. This primary pulmonary vein extends towards the developing lung buds, establishing contact with the venous intrapulmonary plexus and allowing drainage toward the left side of the primitive atrium. This sets the stage for the separation of the systemic and pulmonary circulation by atrial septation.

The process commences in the atrioventricular canal with the development of two opposing masses of mesenchymal tissue—the atrioventricular endocardial cushions. These masses are situated at the superior and inferior borders of the atrioventricular canal. After fusing with two lateral atrioventricular cushions, on the right and left borders of the canal, the canal is completely divided. The right and left atrioventricular orifices are completed. At the same time, a crescentic ingrowth develops on the dorsocephalic part (roof) of the primitive atrium, towards the left of the commissure of the valves of the sinus venosus. This growth, known as the *septum primum*, descends through the cavity of the primitive atrium. As it approaches the fusing endocardial cushions, its development terminates forming the *foramen primum*, a communication between both atrial chambers. With further development of the endocardial cushions and the extension of the atrioventricular septum, the *foramen primum* closes. At the same time, the upper edge of the septum disintegrates, establishing the *ostium secundum*. This ensures free blood flow between both primitive atria. The *septum primum* grows in close apposition and fuses with the left valve of the *sinus venosus*. The fused left atrial valve produces the inferior limbus of the interatrial septum; the right atrial valve; the Eustachian and Thebesian valves. About the time that the secondary interatrial opening is formed and the right atrium expands as it incorporates the sinus horn, a new secondary fold appears between the orifice of the cardial veins (superior vena

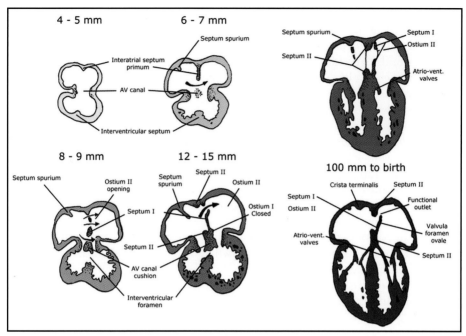

Figure 7. Sections of heart at various developmental periods (Frontal)—4-5 mm (26–27 days); 6–7 mm (30–31 days); 8-9 mm (32-34 days); 12–15 mm (±37 days); 25-30 mm (±50 days); and 100 mm to birth (±14 weeks to birth) (Patten, 1953).

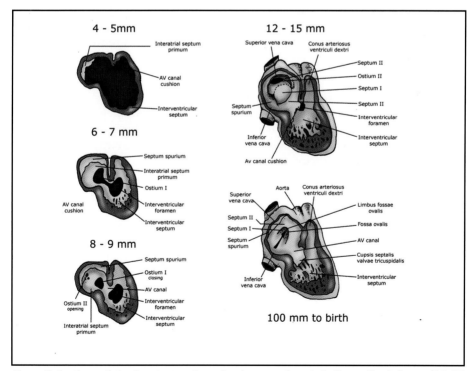

Figure 8. Sections of the heart at various developmental periods (Lateral)—4–5 mm (26–27 days); 6–7 mm (30–31 days); 8–9 mm (32–34 days); 12–15 mm (±37 days); 25–30 mm (±50 days); and 100 mm to birth (±14 weeks to birth) (Patten, 1953).

cava), and the primary pulmonary vein. When the left sinus valve and the *septum spurium* fuse with the right side of the *septum secundum,* a free concave edge of the *septum secundum* starts to overlap the ostium secundum. The *crescentic septum* extends towards the atrioventricular canal to form the upper limbus of the *foramen ovale* although it never quite separates the atrial cavity, leaving an oval aperture. Folding of the edges produces a "doorframe" into which the *septum primum*, in adults named the valvula *foramen ovale*, can shut and, with this, the *foramen ovale* is formed.

Further changes occur within the newly formed left atrium. The primary pulmonary vein loses its initial contact with the splanchnic venous plexus of the foregut. This definitive separation of the foregut enables pulmonary venous return to enter the left atrium. The left atrium is then able to increase in size by integrating the primary pulmonary vein and the first branches of the intrapulmonary veins on either side into the posterior left atrial wall. In the fully developed heart, the original left heart is represented by little more than the trabeculated atrial appendage, while the smooth walled part originates from the pulmonary veins.

The development and division of the ventricles are irrelevant to embryology of the PFO and consequently not included in this work.

COURSE AND BALANCE OF BLOOD FLOW IN THE FETAL AND IN THE NEONATAL HEART

Some knowledge of the changes in the cardiocirculatory system at birth is essential to understand the function of the atria and the anatomical implications of certain embryological structures in the adult. Accordingly, in the next section we review the functional anatomy of the interatrial septum in the fetal and adult stages.

BLOOD FLOW IN THE FETAL HEART

While in utero, the fetal atria are never fully separated. Three communications permit the left atrium to receive blood from the inferior caval vein throughout prenatal life. The greater transseptal flow compensates for the rudimentary pulmonary circulation so that a circulatory balance of the right and left sides of the heart is maintained.

The technical difficulties in gaining access to the fetus in utero have prevented a careful study of flow patterns. Manipulation of a living fetus also disturbs normal physiological functions making it nearly impossible to measure blood flow and pressure with any accuracy.

In 1941 Barcroft, Barron and co workers were the first to obtain blood samples and measure oxygen tension in different localized samples of the fetal circulation (Patten, 1953). In 1944 Barclay and Franklin used contrast angiography to study dynamic fetal circulation more closely (Patten, 1953). Their methods are still in use today and have led to the following model: blood entering the inferior caval entrance, assisted by its valve, is directed towards the foramen ovale, thereby guiding a major portion of the blood flow transseptally into the left atrium.

Blood originating from the inferior caval vein varies considerably in oxygen content with time. The placental blood mixes with deoxygenated blood returning from the lower limbs. A sphincter mechanism in the ductus venosus, where the umbilical vein joins the portal vein, regulates the blood flow entering the right atrium. The sphincter probably constricts during uterine contraction, preventing a sudden overload of the heart due to high venous pressure. During this period, blood originating from the systemic and portal vessels is depleted of oxygen. When the sphincter relaxes, placental oxygenated blood surges towards the right atrium as the blood accumulation is released.

A small portion of the inferior caval blood flow is retained within the right atrium by the lower edge of the *septum secundum*. Blood entering the right atrium from the superior caval vein, is directed downwards through the tricuspid valve into the right ventricle. This blood is mainly deoxygenated; it comes from the head region and is pumped into the pulmonary artery by the right ventricle. It passes through the *ductus arteriosus* into the descending aorta and through the two umbilical veins into the placenta.

During these developments, there is a continuous readjustment of the circulatory flow. As pulmonary blood flow increases, so atrial transseptal flow decreases. Very early in the development, while the lung buds are still connected to the splanchnic plexus, the pulmonary return is small and the flow from the right atrium through the interatrial *ostium primum* constitutes practically the entire intake of the left atrium. In the latter part of fetal life, when the lungs grow rapidly, a progressively smaller part of the left atrial intake comes by way of the foramen ovale. The larger amount of blood comes from the growing lungs, now isolated from the splanchnic circulation.

BLOOD FLOW IN THE NEONATAL HEART

Following birth, there is an abrupt loss of placental circulation and an immediate increase in the pulmonary circulation. All these changes in blood balance and vascular resistance have to accommodated by the heart. As the systemic vascular resistance increases, there is a dramatic increase in aortic pressure, as well as pressure increases in the left ventricle (Guyton, 1981). In contrast, the pulmonary vascular resistance decreases five-fold as a function of expansion of the blood vessels and the loss of hypoxic vasoconstriction (Guyton, 1981). This consequently reduces the pulmonary arterial pressure as well as the right atrial and ventricular pressure.

The pressure reversal between left (high) and right (low) atria leads to a tendency for blood to flow back into the right atrium—in the opposite direction of fetal blood flow. However, the design of the *valvula foramina ovalis*, lying over the foramen, is such that it acts like a one-way valve: it is permissive of right-to-left flow but prevents left-to-right flow. Over time, there is an increase in connective tissue, and the valve and septum become more rigid until all that remains is a slit, which is no longer functional, even though it is probe-patent (Patten, 1953). In two-thirds of the population the valve becomes adherent to the septum and closes permanently. However, even if such closure does not occur, the elevated left atrial pressure (which is 2–4 mm Hg higher than right atrial pressure) retains closure of the valve (Guyton, 1981). Patten has also emphasized that this does not represent a functional handicap in an otherwise normal individual (Patten, 1931, 1953). Sadler suggested that crying spells during the first days of life, may result in right to left shunting (Sadler, 1990b; Sadler and Langman, 2000, 2004); Hoffman suggested the ultimate closure may occur only after several years (Hoffman et al., 1965). Nadas and Fyler wrote that ongoing right-to-left shunt only occurred in cases of obstruction of the right ventricle, pulmonary valves, or due to high pulmonary vascular resistance (Nadas and Fyler, 1972).

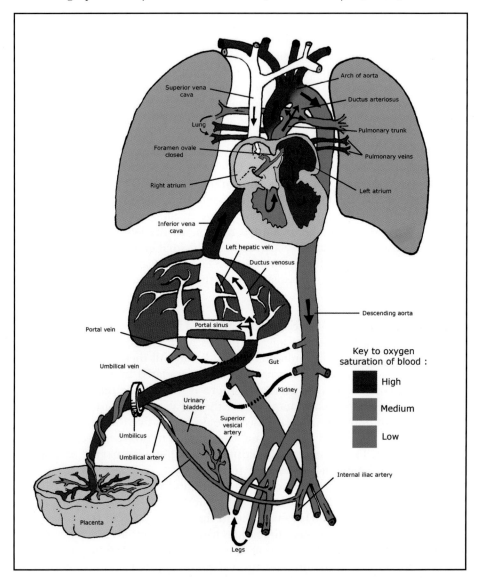

Figure 9. Blood flow in the fetal heart. Three shunts permit most of the blood to bypass the liver and the lungs: (1) the ductus venosus, (2) the foramen ovale, and (3) the ductus arteriosus. A sphincter mechanism in the ductus venosus, where the umbilical vein joins the portal vein, regulates the blood flow to the right atrium (Moore 1988).

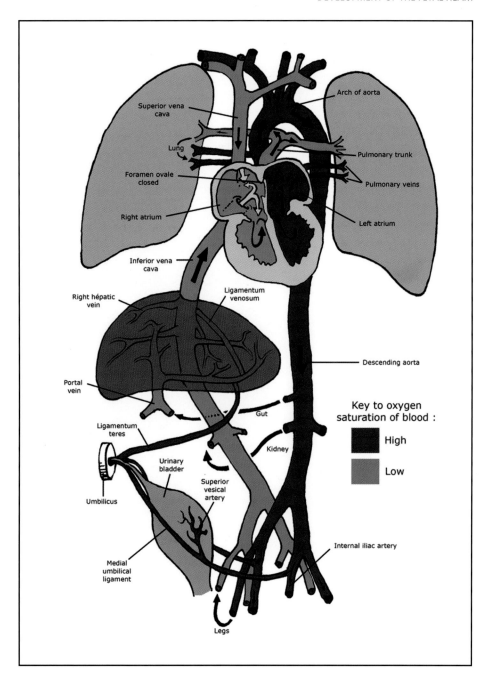

Figure 10. Blood flow after birth. As generally, described, after birth, the three shunts that short-circuited the blood during fetal life cease to function, and the pulmonary and systemic circulations become separated. The adult derivates of the fetal vessels and structures that become nonfunctional at birth are also represented (Moore, 1988).

NOTES

CHAPTER 4

Paradoxical Nitrogen Bubble Embolization Through A PFO: A Cause of DCI in Sport Divers?

INTRODUCTION

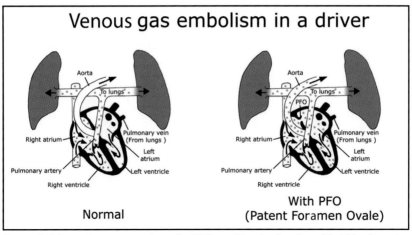

Figure 1. Schematic representation of a PFO resulting in shunting of bubbles from the right to the left side of the heart—i.e., paradoxical gas embolization.

Exposure to inert† gas (i.e., nitrogen or helium) under pressure predisposes divers to problems during and after they return to the surface after a dive. Generally, it is accepted that decompression illness (DCI) is caused by the formation of inert gas bubbles in the venous blood and supersaturated body tissues.

---

† Compressed gas diving beyond 6 to 8 meters requires the addition of inert gas to avoid oxygen toxicity. For practical and economical reasons compressed air and nitrox (i.e., oxygen and nitrogen mixtures different to air) are usually used to depths of 40 to 50 meters. At this point, however, nitrogen narcosis becomes a significant hazard and non-narcotic helium is typically added to the breathing mixture (i.e., trimix). Ultimately, at extreme depths breathing resistance and high pressure nervous syndrome (HPNS) become troublesome and rates of compression and titrations of narcotic nitrogen and non-narcotic, low-density helium (and even hydrogen) have been used to walk the physiological tightrope between ventilatory failure, gas toxicity and HPNS. Importantly, all gases that are not metabolized by the body can cause decompression illness. These are collectively called inert gases. Being the major constituent of air and nitrox, nitrogen is the most common inert gas in recreational diving. However, references to nitrogen—in the context of decompression—also apply to other inert gases unless otherwise specified.

DCI caused by the traumatic intravasation of pulmonary gas due to pulmonary barotrauma (PB) causes AGE that does not involve cardiac shunting and so lies largely outside our current consideration.

Although many factors affect the formation, migration, and reaction to bubbles in the body (Carturan, 1999; Carturan et al., 1999), the risk for developing DCI is related to the extent of the inert gas exposure (saturation) and the rate of ascent (decompression) (Gardette, 1979; Eckenhoff et al., 1990).

Decompression "rules" have been developed that, when followed, offer reasonable protection from DCI. Nevertheless, DCI occurs in sports divers even after uneventful dives and without any overt violations in decompression procedures. In fact it has been shown that even when these rules are followed, nitrogen bubbles can be present in central venous blood in large enough quantities to cause DCI (Buhlmann, 1975; Marroni and Zannini, 1981; Broome, 1996).

The prevailing understanding is that most venous gas bubbles embolize the pulmonary vasculature and are largely "filtered out" following a short period of blockage. Thus, the lung acts as an efficient "bubble filter" (Butler and Hills, 1979) and, under normal conditions, this mechanism would only fail if the number of bubbles delivered into the pulmonary circulatory system is excessive (Vik et al., 1990). This is one of the important reasons why bubble production should be minimized (Egi and Gurmen, 2000), and "low-bubble" decompression schedules should be used (Uguccioni et al., 1995); this is also one of the important research areas being explored by Divers Alert Network (DAN) Europe (Marroni et al., 2001c, 2001b; Marroni et al., 2002b).

Arterialization of venous gas emboli may occur via a PFO in the heart (Crook, 1977; Vik et al., 1993; Reul et al., 1995; Gerriets et al., 2000). Indeed, serious decompression illness—particularly cerebral and high spinal DCI—following innocuous dives, has been associated with the presence of a PFO. This condition is present in 25–30% of all humans, as a remainder of the fetal cardiac anatomy (Hagen et al., 1984).

PFO is a potential right-to-left atrial shunt that may open in response to changes in the interatrial pressure balance—when the right atrial pressure exceeds that of the left—such as may follow the release of prolonged straining maneuvers where there has been a significant increase in intrathoracic pressure.

Importantly, PFO does not result in a continuous passage of blood between the right and the left atrium. The reason for this is as follows: Firstly, the atrial pressure on the right side of the heart is generally (i.e., in 95% of the duration of the cardiac cycle) lower than on the left side. Secondly, the Foramen Ovale is a one-way valve that only opens when right atrial pressure exceeds left atrial pressure (Cambier et al., 1993). Thirdly, the blood enters the heart from both the superior and inferior vena cavae. This leads to venous turbulence in the right atrium, which tends to sweep bubbles away from the interatrial septum. Accordingly blood coming from the inferior vena cava (which would contain most of the decompression nitrogen bubbles) is diverted away from the PFO (Gin et al., 1993). These three mechanisms are natural barriers to paradoxical embolism through a PFO.

After diving, however, two factors may facilitate right-to-left shunting. Continuous pulmonary embolization of nitrogen microbubbles will ultimately lead to an increase in pulmonary vascular resistance. This may increase right atrial pressure to the point that it allows shunting of blood (Vik et al., 1993).

In addition, as has been clearly demonstrated during contrast trans-esophageal echocardiography (c-TEE), certain respiratory maneuvers may cause a temporary reversal of interatrial pressures and thus permit shunting. These maneuvers are detailed in another chapter and can be voluntary or involuntary (Cambier et al., 1993; Balestra et al., 1998).

PFO can thus be responsible for some of the so-called "unexplained" or "unpredictable" forms of DCI, especially the cerebral, high-spinal and cutaneous varieties. The estimated "Odds Ratio" for DCI when diving with a PFO ranges from 2.5 (Bove, 1998) to 4.5 for cerebral-type DCI (Germonpre et al., 1998a).

STUDY PROTOCOL

To examine the possible correlation between PFO and certain forms of neurological and audio-vestibular decompression illness, the authors performed a study involving Belgian divers who had suffered neurological DCI during the period 1991–1995; they had been treated in either the Ostend Naval Hospital or Brussels Military Hospital Hyperbaric Centers. The study protocol was approved by the Ethics Committees of the respective institutions, and informed consent was obtained from all subjects.

The exclusion criteria were:
- Uncertainty in the diagnosis of DCI
- Unreliable dive profile reporting
- Voluntary withdrawal from the study
- Evidence of cardiac or pulmonary disease at the time of the investigation.

DCI is a relatively rare complication of SCUBA diving. Only 30 cases are reported annually in Belgium. Frequently the symptoms are minor, vague, and subjective, so that the diagnosis becomes ambiguous. Lack of response to recompression introduces additional doubt. On the other hand, rapid onset of neurological symptoms following a dive is highly suspicious of DCI. Over the study period, nearly 50% of all cases had to be excluded due to uncertainty of diagnosis

Cerebral air embolism, arising from microscopic pulmonary barotrauma, has been described as a possible cause of unexplained DCI (Wilmshurst et al., 1989). Although it is not possible to rule out this diagnosis with certainty, those cases where this was considered likely, were rejected. By carefully performing a clinical examination and reviewing the dive profile, all the cases where pulmonary barotrauma was still a possibility, were subjected to high-resolution computed tomography and spirometry testing (i.e., including flow-volume loops). The divers were included only if these examinations revealed no abnormalities. Thirteen divers were excluded on this basis. Part of the workup included transthoracic echocardiography (TTE) which allowed the evaluation of possible occult pulmonary hypertension. None of the subjects showed evidence of pulmonary hypertension (i.e., pulmonary artery acceleration time <120 msec, maximal velocity of regurgitant tricuspid flow—when present—below 2.5m/sec) or any sign of cardiac dysfunction). Other exclusion criteria included:

- Unreliable dive profile reporting—such as inconsistencies in the diver's history—led to the exclusion of 20% of cases.
- Voluntary withdrawal from the study. Six divers refused trans-esophageal echocardiography (TEE) and withdrew from the study.
- Evidence of cardiac or pulmonary disease at the time of the investigation.

Intermittent diving activity or a history of previous DCI were not considered grounds for exclusion.

Eventually 37 divers with neurological DCI were included. According to their symptoms, they were classified as having suffered from:

- "Spinal" DCI—uni- or bi-lateral lower extremity paresthesia, paresis or paralysis, bladder or bowel dysfunction, or a combination of these, often with mid-dorsal pain as the first presenting symptom, or
- "Cerebral" DCI—cerebral, cerebellar, high-spinal, vestibular or cochlear symptoms).

The following dive profile characteristics were recorded: dive depth; bottom time; single or repetitive dive; computer or dive tables used; inclusion or omission of any safety or decompression stops; and the presence of rapid ascents. "Minor" risk factors were also noted, such as pre-dive fatigue, stress, alcohol consumption; dehydration (inadequate fluid intake); physical exertion; feeling of cold during the dive; and post-dive exercise. A DCI episode was classified as "unexplained" when no errors had been made in ascent rate or decompression stops; a maximum of three "minor" risk factors were also accepted.

For each participating diver, a matched control diver was selected from the Belgian diving population—one who had never suffered DCI. Matching criteria included the following: age (±5years); gender; body mass index (BMI; weight/(height)2: ±2 kg/m²); smoking habits (classified into three categories according to the number of pack-years (PY) smoked: <5 PY, 5–10 PY or >10 PY); physical condition as judged by diver and examiner (roughly estimated as bad, moderate or good); diving experience (number of years diving, total number of dives, ±10%); and Eustachian tube patency (i.e., need for vigorous Valsalva maneuver vs. other methods of ear equalization)[†]. Thirty-six control divers were finally selected.

All divers underwent TEE with the use of agitated saline bubble contrast. In brief, TEE was performed by means of a multiplane echocardiographic probe (HP Sonos 2500), in the awake or mildly sedated patient. The interatrial septum was located and the ultrasound probe positioned to allow a clear view of both right and left atrium. Via an antebrachial vein perfusion, agitated saline (9.5 mL saline and 0.5mL air, pushed back and forth ten times in a double syringe system to promote cavitation) was rapidly injected to provide contrast. Correct injection of this volume resulted in a massive opacification of the right atrium. The number of bubbles appearing in the left atrium within three heart cycles after complete opacification of the right atrium was noted.

After at least two injections, each with a one-minute interval in order to clear the right atrium completely of remaining bubbles, the patient was asked

---

† Anticipating the hypothesis that diving and/or repeated Valsalva maneuvers could be associated with a failure to fuse or result in secondary re-opening of a Foramen Ovale we also selected control divers based on years of diving experience and ear equalization method used (see Discussion).

to perform a high-strain Valsalva maneuver, which was held for approximately ten seconds before release. Agitated saline was injected during this maneuver. At the arrival of the first bubbles in the right atrium, the patient was instructed to release the strain. This resulted in a brisk leftward bulging of the interatrial septum. Again, any passage of bubbles to the left atrium was noted.

This contrast TEE (C-TEE) method was applied in a strictly standardized fashion by two experienced cardiologists. All c-TEE's were recorded onto high-resolution videotape (super-VHS) and reviewed at a later stage by both cardiologists together in a blinded manner. Bubble counts were performed manually on high-quality still-frame video images. Care was taken to exclude spontaneous respiratory contrast (Van Camp et al. 1994).

Patency of the Foramen Ovale was classified into three grades (see Figure 2):

- **Grade 0:** no contrast passage at rest or after Valsalva strain
- **Grade I:** no or slight (<20 bubbles) contrast passage at rest or after Valsalva strain
- **Grade II:** important (>20 bubbles) contrast passage at rest or after Valsalva strain

Statistical Analysis

The results were analyzed by means of a standard statistical software package on IBM PC (SPSS 6 for Windows). The null hypothesis was that there would be no difference in PFO prevalence between DCI divers and

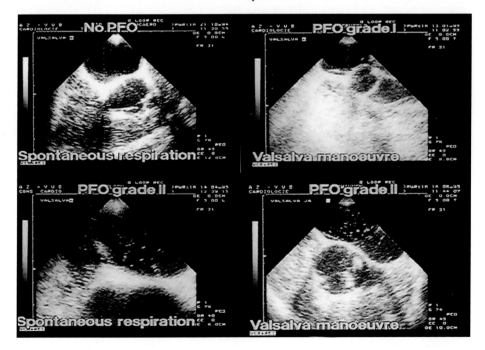

Figure 2. Classification of PFO Grades:
Grade 0: no contrast passage at rest or after Valsalva strain
Grade I: no or slight (<20 bubbles) contrast passage at rest or after Valsalva strain
Grade II: important (>20 bubbles) contrast passage at rest or after Valsalva strain

control divers in any of the subgroups. P-values were calculated using Fisher's exact test. Biometric and dive data were analyzed using Student's unpaired t-test, or Fischer's exact test where appropriate.

RESULTS

The overall prevalence of PFO in DCI divers was 22/37 (59.5%) marginally, though not statistically, higher than in the matched controls divers: 13/36 (36.1%, p=0.06). However, in the subgroup of divers with cerebral DCI, the prevalence of PFO was significantly higher than in matched controls (16/20 vs. 5/20; p=0.012), whereas in the subgroup of divers with spinal DCI the PFO prevalence was comparable to the matched controls with no statistically significant difference (6/17 vs. 8/16; p=0.49).

For Grade II PFO's, the difference between those with cerebral DCI and matched controls was even greater (14/20 vs. 3/20; p=0.002), whereas the spinal DCI subgroup still did not reach statistical significance compared to matched controls (5/17 vs. 6/16; p=0.29).

To exclude confounding factors related to dive depth these were specifically analyzed (Table 4-2). No significant differences were found, although cerebral DCI tended to occur at shallower depths. Fourteen out of 17 spinal DCI cases could be classified as "unexplained" compared to 12 out of 20 cerebral DCI cases (p=0.17).

The number of divers using dive computers vs. dive tables to plan their dives was not statistically different. Computer divers in the cerebral DCI and spinal DCI subgroups generally performed deeper dives, but these differences were not statistically significant.

Divers with spinal DCI tended to dive slightly deeper than divers with cerebral DCI. Time to onset of symptoms tended to be longer in the spinal DCI group.

With regard to the biometric data—age; body mass index (BMI); smoking habits; and the diving experience—no significant differences were found between the spinal and cerebral DCI subgroups (Table 4–3).

However, there was a striking difference in the method used for middle ear equalization. While the spinal DCI subgroup had spontaneous Eustachian

TABLE 1. PREVALENCE OF PFO IN DIVERS WITH DCI

	PFO	%	Grade 2 PFO	%
All DCI	22/37	59.5%	19/37	51.3%
All Controls	13/36	36.1%	9/36	25%
P	0.06		0.03	
Cerebral DCI	16/20	80%	14/20	70%
Matched Controls	5/20	25%	3/20	15%
P	0.012		0.002	
Spinal DCI	6/17	35.2%	5/17	29.4%
Matched Control	8/16	50%	6/16	37.5%
P	0.49		0.29	

TABLE 2. ANALYSIS OF DIVES LEADING TO DCI

	N	Dive Depth (m)	Computer (mean depth, m)	Tables (mean depth, m)	Unexplained vs. All DCI	Symptom onset (min)
Cerebral	20	35±11	10/20 (37.4±10.2)	10/20 (31.4±10.1)	12/20	32±48
Spinal	17	41±8	6/17 (45.0±8.8)	11/17 (39.0±6.8)	14/17	79±187
P		0.07	0.15	0.06	0.17	0.33

m=meters sea water; min=minutes

Tube Patency (ETP) in 8/17 divers (i.e., they had no difficulties for equalizing middle ear pressure by yawning or only very light Valsalva maneuver), *all* the divers from the cerebral DCI subgroup reported they had to "push hard" or "push really hard" to clear their ears while diving (p=0.006).

Finally, we looked at those divers with "unexplained" DCI (26/37, 70.3%). In the cerebral DCI group (n=12), one had a PFO Grade I and ten had Grade II (10/12, 83%). In the spinal DCI subgroup (n= 14), two had PFO Grade I and 4 had Grade II (6/14, 43%). The association of unexplained DCI and PFO was borderline significant for all types of PFO (p=0.05) and statistically significant for Grade II PFO (p=0.047).

Considering all divers who suffered DCI, divers with PFO had a significantly higher prevalence of PFO (16/22, 73%) than divers without PFO (4/15, 26%) (p=0.0084); even for PFO Grade II alone, this was still statistically significant (14/19 vs. 6/18, p=0.021). The Odds Ratio for cerebral DCI with PFO was 7.33 (all PFO's) and 5.6 (PFO Grade II), respectively.

DISCUSSION

PFO is present in about 30% of the normal population; the prevalence seems to decline with ascending age (Hagen et al., 1984). The anatomical details of PFO are well known: in most cases it consists of a narrow (1–6 mm), rather long (7 mm) channel, traversing the interatrial septum from upper

TABLE 3. BIOMETRIC DATA OF THE DCI POPULATION

	N	Age	BMI	Smokers >10 PY	Dive Years	Dives	ETP
Cerebral	20	37±9	26±4	8/20	8±6	327±282	0/20
Spinal	17	38±9	45±8.8	4/17	12±10	481±465	8/17
P		0.59	0.36	0.32	0.16	0.25	0.006

BMI:weight/(height)^2; PY:pack-year; ETP: Eustachian Tube Patency

TABLE 4. SENSITIVITY AND SPECIFICITY OF DIFFERENT ECHODOPPLER PFO DETECTION †

	c-Tee		c-TTe		Carotid Doppler		c-TCD	
	Sens.	Spec.	Sens.	Spec.	Sens.	Spec.	Sens.	Spec.
Blatteau, 1999					100%	88%		
Belkin, et al., 1994			50%	92%				
Schneider et al., 1996	89%	100%						
Di Tullio et al.,1993b			47%	100%			68%	100%
Job et al., 1994							89%	92%
Klotzsch et al., 1994							91.5%	93.8%
Chimowitz et al., 1991	100%	100%	54%	94%			100%	100%
Jauss et al., 1994	93%	100%						
Heckmann et al., 1999	92.3%	100%					84.6%	100%

right posterior to lower left anterior (Cambier et al., 1993). Thus, it forms a functional valve through which, under normal hemodynamic conditions, no significant blood shunt occurs; the right atrial pressure is usually lower than the left atrial pressure maintaining closure of the one-way valve. In some patients, a reversal of the pressure gradient may transiently occur in the cardiac cycle, but unless there is a very wide opening, no significant shunting occurs (Strunk et al., 1987). If a persistent left-to right shunt is present, the term "PFO" is no longer appropriate, and the term "atrial septal defect" (ASD) should be applied.

ASD, although mostly asymptomatic, is an established contra-indication for sports diving, whereas PFO is not considered a contra-indication by most diving medical experts.

During recent years, several clinical studies have indicated the possibility of a higher prevalence of PFO in divers who have suffered from DCI (Moon et al., 1989; Wilmshurst et al., 1989). These authors concluded that PFO could be the cause of DCI by way of permitting paradoxical embolism of nitrogen bubbles that may otherwise have been filtered out by the lung vasculature. In the absence of a decompression error, a PFO might explain the cause of otherwise "unexplained" DCI. This hypothesis has subsequently been challenged (Smith et al., 1990a, 1990b; Cross et al., 1992).

All these authors used contrast transthoracic echocardiography (c-TTE) to diagnose PFO, even though TEE is known to be more sensitive (Siostrzonek et al., 1991). However, TEE is more invasive and compliance is affected accordingly. Transcranial Doppler (TCD) has been used increasingly in recent years, but has reduced sensitivity due to the inability to distinguish between PFO and trans-pulmonary shunting.

† For the purposes of diving sensitivity and specificity, c-TEE was compared to cardiac catheterization whereas other methods were compared to c-TEE.

From the above it is conceivable that several significant PFO's may have been "missed" using TTE. Also, the contrast and Valsalva technique may have had a negative impact on PFO detection.

Valsalva maneuvers are commonly employed to enhance the sensitivity of contrast echocardiography. The goal, by augmenting the intrathoracic pressure (ITP), is to obstruct the venous inflow temporarily. Upon release of the intrathoracic pressure, the inflow of pooled blood causes a significant rise in the right atrial pressure. This may consequently sweep saline bubbles towards the interatrial septal and through a PFO. Importantly, however, contrast generation, injection and Valsalva maneuvers must be timed and performed correctly. Otherwise, the right atria do not opacify at the time of right atrial pressure reversal nor will contrast reach the interatrial septum— the result being a false negative study. Owing to natural flow patterns in the right atrium, contrast should be injected into a large lower extremity vein ideally, but this is usually impractical. Complete opacification of the right atrium is therefore an important quality control measure during echocardiographic assessment of PFO.

In another chapter, we consider the details of intrathoracic pressure (ITP) in relation to PFO evaluation. Of importance here is that we have been able to demonstrate that the slope of ITP reduction is independent of the technique used (Marroni and Balestra, 1996; Balestra et al., 1998). On the other hand, to augment TEE sensitivity effectively, the *duration* of the increase in ITP is extremely important. A simple cough, although achieving a high ITP (Stoddard et al., 1993), does not last long enough to be truly effective. It would only be better than a Valsalva maneuver if the latter were improperly performed or insufficiently sustained.

In our study, the prevalence of PFO in the control divers was higher than reported in autopsy studies (Hagen et al., 1984; Vandenbogaerde et al., 1992; Cambier et al., 1993). This may be a coincidental finding, but there is also lingering uncertainty whether PFO size and patency remains static in adult life: The declining prevalence of PFO with advancing age suggests a gradual secondary adhesion and solidification of the two leaflets. On the other hand, the size of persistent shunts tends to increase (Hagen et al., 1984; Sacco et al., 1993). We consider the possible implications of this phenomenon in detail in another chapter.

While still subject to debate, it appears as though PFO-related DCI symptoms usually appear very shortly (less than 30 minutes) after the dive (Wilmshurst et al., 1989). Surprisingly, even though hemodynamic considerations would predict preferential embolization of cerebral or high spinal regions, this has not been confirmed definitively (Wilmshurst et al., 1994). This has led the authors to postulate that the development of cerebral DCI may be related to mechanisms other than simple paradoxical nitrogen bubble embolization.

Finally, our study included an exceptionally high number of "unexplained" DCI (26/37, 70.3%). Typically, "undeserved" or "unexplained" DCI makes up 40–50% DCI. However, we excluded all but the most definite manifestations following well-reported dive profiles. This undoubtedly affected the results by excluding both possible, but atypical, and doubtful cases. On the other hand, the manifestations that were retained for investigation were those representing the areas of greatest concern—unambiguous, significant, neurological impairment.

CONCLUSIONS

Our study supports a significant correlation between the prevalence of PFO and the occurrence of cerebral but not spinal DCI. This is consistent with a pathophysiological model in which nitrogen bubbles, passing through a PFO into the arterial circulation, subsequently migrate preferentially towards the carotid and/or vertebral arteries. Accordingly, within the defined scope and limitations of the methodology employed, this study supports the hypothesis that patency of a Foramen Ovale is associated with cerebral DCI where pulmonary barotraumatic arterial gas embolism has been reasonably excluded as an alternative cause.

We recommend that divers with unexplained DCI, particularly with cerebral or high-spinal localization, be examined for the presence of a PFO particularly if they intend returning to diving or suffer from recurrent migraine[†] (Lechat et al., 1989; Bogousslavsky et al., 1996; Anzola et al., 1999; Cujec et al., 1999; Anzola et al., 2000; Wahl et al., 2001; Lamy et al., 2002a; Lamy et al., 2002b; Sztajzel et al., 2002).

If a Grade II PFO is present, paradoxical nitrogen bubble embolization is more likely and we would advise the diver who wishes to continue diving, to (1) take every precaution to reduce the number of circulating venous gas emboli after a dive and (2) to avoid Valsalva maneuvers during ascent and for at least two hours after reaching the surface.

Furthermore, for future PFO studies, we strongly recommend:

- using a standardized c-TEE technique, with special attention to the strain and duration of the Valsalva maneuver
- semi-quantifying the patency of the Foramen Ovale
- using matched divers as controls

---

† Recurrent migraine has been associated with the presence of PFO and ASD; it also carries a greater risk of subsequent ischemic stroke irrespective of an diving activity and may accordingly justify medical intervention.

CHAPTER 5

CAN WE DEFINE THE RELATIVE RISK OF INCURRING DCI RELATED TO THE PRESENCE OF A PFO?

INTRODUCTION

Retrospective studies do not permit the calculation of relative risk (Laupacis et al., 1988).

Odds ratios may be determined, however, and there is indeed a relationship between the two. If a disease is rare (i.e., less than a few percent of the population studied), then the odds ratio will be comparable to relative risk (Motulsky, 1995). DCI has an incidence rate of four per 10,000 dives and thus meets this requirement.

If applying this principle to our study, the following would be found in calculating the odds ratio for PFO's using the Fisher's exact test.

INCIDENCE OF PFO GRADE II
IN ALL DECOMPRESSION ILLNESSES

According to Fisher's Exact Test:
The two-sided P value is 0.0301—statistically significant.
The row/column association is statistically significant.
Odds ratio=3.167 (95% Confidence Interval: 1.174 to 8.544)

TABLE 1. DATA ANALYZED ACCORDING TO FISHER'S TEST

	DCI	No DCI	TOTAL
PFO2	(A) 19	(B) 9	28
No PFO	(C) 18	(D) 27	45
TOTAL	37	36	73

If, by applying Motulsky's principle, we reanalyze our data to determine relative risk, this would be done as follows:

$$RR = \dfrac{\dfrac{A}{A+B}}{\dfrac{C}{C+D}} \qquad \text{the odds will be: } OR = \dfrac{\dfrac{A}{B}}{\dfrac{C}{D}}$$

The resulting "relative risk" would therefore be 1.7 whereas the odds ratio is 3.4.

The difference is important, particularly when considering the amplitude of the 95% confidence interval and the potential impact if the (A) value had been smaller. In any event, the data of the study at least, does not support applying Motulsky's approximation for PFO (Motulsky, 1995).

To overcome this challenge, we decided to perform: (1) a prospective study with, (2) a large patient sample, using, (3), an ethical, acceptable, minimally invasive and reliable test for PFO screening, that had been, (4) validated using a accepted gold standard investigation with, (5) a standardized contrast and Valsalva maneuver.

Before embarking on the study, the appropriate test procedure had to be developed first, as outlined in chapter entitled, "Carotid Artery Doppler as a Minimally Invasive Screening Method for PFO."

CHAPTER 6

CAROTID ARTERY DOPPLER AS A MINIMALLY INVASIVE SCREENING METHOD FOR PFO (CORRELATION WITH C-TEE)

INTRODUCTION

Patent Foramen Ovale (PFO) has been associated with DCI in divers. The proposed mechanism is arterialization of venous gas (i.e., paradoxical nitrogen bubble embolization). It is suspected when conservative dives result in severe DCI but the dive history and physical findings do not support the possibility of pulmonary barotrauma. Previous studies suggest that there is a significant correlation between cerebral DCI and the presence of a large PFO (i.e., Grade II or >20 bubbles shunting through the interatrial septum, in the absence of an atrial septal defect, during a single cardiac cycle) (Moon et al., 1989; Wilmshurst et al., 1989; Germonpre et al., 1998b). The association between PFO and so-called "undeserved DCI" is statistically significant, given that the evidence is based on a relatively small number of individuals (approximately 100 individuals) and are all retrospective studies. To date no prospective studies have been published. Recently, a further attempt was made to establish relative risk (Torti et al., 2004). Although a large population was studied, this study suffered from a number of shortcomings so that it did not provide a definitive answer (Germonpre and Balestra, 2004).

Studying the relationship between PFO and DCI is complicated by the relatively low incidence of the latter (i.e., approximately one case of DCI per 10,000 dives). This means that—for the purposes of a useful prospective study—a large number of divers would need to be screened. Assuming the divers perform 100 dives per year, 2,000 divers would need to be examined in order to observe approximately 20 cases of DCI. Dangerous, costly or very invasive investigations would be inappropriate. For these reasons c-TEE—the gold standard—would be impractical; a more convenient screening method would be required. To be effective, screening would need to be:

- easy to perform by a general medical practitioner/physician (and therefore possibly be included in annual dive fitness examination)
- simple, require minimal assistance, and not be time-consuming
- tolerated by study participants
- inexpensive

Carotid Doppler (c-CD) with bubble contrast (c-CD) meets these requirements. Given the right specificity and sensitivity, it would therefore be a useful research tool for screening large quantities of divers.

Several TEE studies have indicated that there is a good correlation between c-TEE and c-CD, but no formal validation has been done until now (Bussiere et al., 1992; Augusseau et al., 1997). The following study aimed to validate c-CD as a means of detecting paradoxical bubble embolization through a PFO.

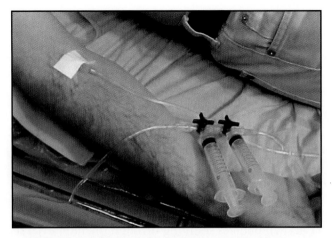

Figure 1. Testing Procedures: Syringe system to produce contrast.

METHODS

The study was designed as a prospective, semi-blinded comparison between early Doppler signal detection in the carotid artery after injection of bubble contrast in a large antebrachial vein, and a subsequent c-TEE examination for detection and semi quantification of a PFO—if present.

Cardiology patients, who required c-TEE for other reasons, were approached regarding willingness to participate in this comparative study. Exclusion criteria included patients with cardiac failure, gross cardiac abnormalities, as well as those requiring sedation or being otherwise unable to perform abdominal straining/Valsalva maneuvers (Balestra et al., 1996; Balestra et al., 1998).

Prior to commencing the study, a large bore venous catheter was placed in an antebrachial vein and connected to a three way valve system; two 10cc syringes attached to the bowels; and a 500cc saline infusion.

Carotid Doppler was performed using a vascular 8 MHz Doppler probe. Signals were monitored by headphones to avoid disturbing the patient and the TEE operator.

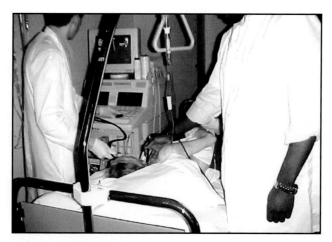

Figure 2. Testing Procedure: Experimental Configuration—simultaneous carotid Doppler and c-TEE.

A good Doppler signal was obtained from the common carotid artery, and throughout the examination, the probe was held in the correct position by a Doppler assistant.

In the literature, various techniques have been described for microbubble contrast generation using different liquids. One of these techniques consists of vigorously shaking a syringe filled with saline and air and then eliminating the extraneous air and injecting the bubble emulsion (Siostrzonek et al., 1991; Van Camp et al., 1994). Another technique used two syringes connected by a three-way valve and, by performing to-and-fro movements of 9.5cc of saline and 0.5cc of air, an emulsion of cavitation microbubbles is produced and subsequently injected (Di Tullio et al., 1993a; Sacco et al., 1993; Stoddard et al., 1993; Germonpre et al., 1998a; Droste et al., 1999). Recent data from a German team using this method reported consistent results (Droste et al., 2002; Torti et al., 2004). These authors also reported the presence of extracardiac or pulmonary shunts. The authors determined an 11% prevalence of shunts amongst the test of subjects compared to 10% in our study (three out of 33 subjects). They emphasized that the contrast passage, while delayed, was similar to intracardiac shunting.

For the purposes of our study, we also selected the two-syringe configuration. Accordingly, saline bubble contrast was generated by agitating 9.5 mL saline with 0.5 mL air between two 10 mL syringes, and then rapidly injecting it into the vein. The appearance of a short series of "clicks" (i.e., for less than three seconds) in the carotid Doppler signal, within five seconds of the end of the injection, was considered "positive," irrespective of whether it was due to an intracardiac or pulmonary shunt (Figures 3 and 4). Early signals (i.e., less than three seconds from the end of injection) were considered highly suggestive of a PFO. The consistent appearance of late signals (i.e., more than five seconds) were considered highly suggestive of a pulmonary shunt (Figure 4). The maneuver was repeated twice during rest and twice following abdominal straining.

The straining maneuver was performed as follows: the patient was instructed to take a deep breath, and purposely hold it while exerting abdominal

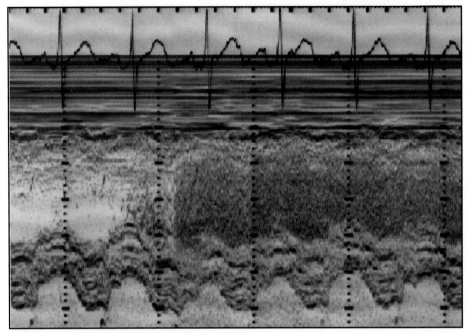

Figure 3. Late contrast passage after Valsalva: pulmonary shunts?

pressure. (Note: to be effective, this maneuver should produce initial bradycardia followed by increasing tachycardia as the maneuver is sustained—these changes are all detectable by Doppler). After ten seconds of straining, the saline bubble contrast was injected. Immediately after the injection, the study participants were asked to exhale and resume normal breathing.

A great deal of importance is given to the proper "straining" technique when doing contrast injections. This straining technique is in fact the "proper" Valsalva maneuver, in contrast to what divers and non-divers consider a Valsalva maneuver to be. In the chapter entitled, "Intrathoracic Pressure Changes after Valsalva Strain and Other Maneuvers: Implications for Divers with PFO," we report on a study performed in 1998 to determine the exact contribution of each of the "straining maneuvers" on intrathoracic pressure rise and fall. The aim was to determine how each of these maneuvers interferes with peripheral (extra-thoracic) blood pooling, and thus determine which of these could potentially enhance right-to-left shunting in divers.

Care was required to ensure that the Doppler probe continued providing a good signal during the maneuvers. For the purposes of blinding, the Doppler assistant was positioned in such a way the results of the TEE scan could not be observed. Similarly, the use of earphones ensured blinding of the Doppler examination (Balestra et al., 2000b).

After this, a standardized contrast TEE examination was performed, as described in an earlier study. The anatomy of the interatrial septum and Fossa Ovalis was then described my means semi quantifying the amount of bubble transfer: Grade 0 (no bubble passage); Grade I (<20 bubbles, either at rest or after straining maneuver); or Grade II (>20 bubbles, either at rest or after straining maneuver). Special attention was given to identify any false

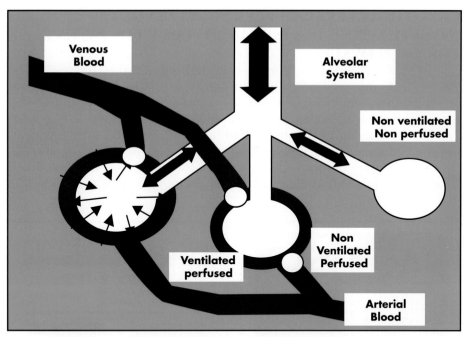

Figure 4. Schematic view of pulmonary shunts.

respiratory contrast (i.e., by performing some straining maneuvers without the injection of contrast either before and after the actual contrast study) whereas "late" contrast appearance, more than four heartbeats after the injection, was attributed to true pulmonary shunts (Torti et al., 2004). These results were analyzed statistically to validate the Doppler methodology in comparison of TEE.

RESULTS

Thirty-three non-diving patients underwent both Doppler and TEE screening methods for PFO. Eight out of the 33 patients were identified as having a PFO using TEE (24%). This is consistent with the normal prevalence. The carotid Doppler (CD) method revealed all eight PFO's (sensitivity: 100%) but yielded three false positive results (specificity: 88%). There were no false negatives. Unlike TEE, CD cannot specifically exclude the pulmonary shunts.

CONCLUSIONS

Although the technique may seem subjective in some respects, C-CD shows excellent sensitivity and specificity when compared to TEE. C-CD may therefore be useful as a low-cost, relatively non-invasive, prospective screening tool for detecting PFO in the diving population. Based on the outcome of this study, we proposed a prospective, multicenter, study to determine the relative risk of PFO in diving. The details of this study are provided in the next section.

CAROTID ARTERY DOPPLER SCREENING: INVESTIGATING DCI RISK IN DIVERS WITH PATENT FORAMEN OVALE

Because of the ongoing interest in determining the risks related to PFO and diving, and following validation of C-CD as an appropriate screening tool, a multicentre, international, prospective study was designed with a projected subject enrollment of 4000 divers to achieve 80% power. Following a number of training workshops in which prospective investigators were trained in the standardized methodology of C-CD a total of 22 investigators were enrolled from Belgium, Italy, Austria, Germany, South Africa, England, and Holland. Between them, they have evaluated 352 divers to date.

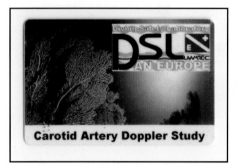 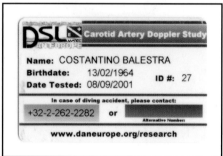

Figure 5 and 6. Sample Card given to every participant.

MATERIAL AVAILABLE ON THE INTERNET

In order to solicit participation in the DAN C-CD Study and to provide reference material, a number of texts have been posted on the DAN Europe Website and are available to divers on *https://www.daneurope.org/eng/english.htm*

After undergoing the screening test, divers receive a plastic card indicating their study participant number and a telephone number.

All over Europe and elsewhere divers have been invited to participate in this study. All that is required from them is their commitment, the time to perform the initial screening assessment, consent to the procedure, and their willingness to report any DCI episodes. This reporting is especially important, as the results are constantly monitored. In case the risk for divers with PFO appears to be unduly high, the study may be terminated before the five-year period, research subjects contacted, and appropriate warnings distributed via DAN to the diving public at large. At the end of the five-year period, each diver will be contacted again by telephone or mail and will be asked how many dives were made in the period and whether there were any DCI incidents. This study protocol was approved by the Ethics Committee of the Belgian Armed Forces on December 8, 2000; and by the Ethics Committee of the NHS Grampian Hospitals, Elgin, Scotland in December 2003.

CHAPTER 7

INTRATHORACIC PRESSURE CHANGES AFTER VALSALVA STRAIN AND OTHER MANEUVERS: IMPLICATIONS FOR DIVERS WITH PFO

INTRODUCTION

SCUBA divers with a PFO may be at risk for paradoxical (right-to-left) nitrogen gas embolization when performing maneuvers that cause a rebound blood loading to the right atrium (Moon et al., 1989). This can cause nitrogen bubbles in the venous blood to be shunted into the left heart and subsequently into the arterial blood flow without transit through the pulmonary circulation where bubble capture could occur. The best-known example of these maneuvers is the Valsalva maneuver (Antonio-Maria Valsalva, 1666–1723), that is commonly used to augment the sensitivity of contrast trans-esophageal echocardiography (c-TEE).

The release of the Valsalva maneuver results in a decrease in airway and intrathoracic pressure (ITP). This is followed by a sudden increase in systemic venous return to the right atrium and an increase in venous filling of the lungs, with a transient decrease in flow into the left heart (Versprille et al., 1982; Cambier et al., 1993). The blood shift resulting from the release of ITP causes a rise in right atrial pressure (RAP) that is easily seen during TEE as a leftward bulging of the interatrial septum. There is also a marked opening of a PFO, if present (Tsai and Chen, 1990; Chen et al., 1992).

It has been suggested that the maneuvers used by divers to equalize the pressure in the middle ear (tympanic) cavity can likewise cause an increase in right atrial pressure and lead to opening of a PFO—if present. Many different maneuvers are employed to equalize the ears. These range from gentle swallowing to a sustained "Valsalva maneuver"—blowing through the blocked nose in order to increase the middle ear pressure by air insufflation of the Eustachian tube. The purpose of the study was to determine if the Valsalva maneuver, as used by divers to equalize the ears, generated similar cardiac changes to the Valsalva straining technique used during c-TEE, and whether the effects on ITP were similar.

METHODS

Sixteen experienced divers (4 females and 12 males) participated in the study. The age range was 22 to 39 years. All subjects consented to the investigation and the experimental methods prior to participation.

We subsequently measured increases and decreases in intrathoracic pressure (ITP) during various maneuvers. ITP pressure changes were measured by means of an 1.5 mL esophageal balloon catheter (filled with saline solution). The balloon was positioned in the lower third of the esophagus (approximately 45 cm from the nostrils in a non-reflexogenic zone). It was then connected to a Marquette TRAM 500 monitoring system (Marquette Electronics, Jupiter, FL 33468, USA) via an Abbott Invasive Blood Pressure Kit (Abbott Laboratories Ltd, Sligo, Rep. of Ireland). The system was calibrated at the level of the xiphoid process. The pressure values obtained were recorded as "relative" pressures, permitting a comparison between values from different maneuvers. The curves were recorded on thermal paper. The test procedures are outlined in Table 1.

TABLE 1. TEST PROCEDURES

1	CONTROL: maximal isometric arm and chest muscle exercises: While sitting in a standard position (i.e., with knees and hips at 90° flexion), arms extended forward in a 90° angle from the chest, the diver had to push down on a scale, placed on the ground, by means of a wooden stick. This test was performed three times; the mean pushdown force was noted, and the mean ITP reached was used as the control ITP value for the other tested maneuvers.
2	GENTLE VALSALVA: Valsalva maneuver (as performed by the divers during the middle ear pressure equalization).
3	FORCED VALSALVA: Valsalva maneuver (maximal): a forced equalizing maneuver.
4	CALIBRATED VALSALVA: Valsalva maneuver (gradually increased until the ITP reached the level of the first maximal isometric exercise).
5	COUGH: forceful coughing.
6	KNEE BEND WITH VALSALVA: knee bend (during breath hold).
7	FREE EXHALING KNEE BEND: knee bend (without breath hold).
8	FINAL ISOMETRIC CONTRACTION: final isometric effort: the diver was instructed to repeat the initial maximal isometric exercise. Care was taken to ensure that the same pushdown force was reached.

The ITP value of the initial isometric muscle exercise was considered to represent 100%, thereby allowing the other maneuvers to be compared to this standard. Next, the slope of the drop in ITP following the maneuver was analyzed to determine the pressure excursion and whether the same peak ITPs could be reached by various maneuvers.

The experimental results were analyzed statistically including mean, standard deviation, median and an analysis of variance (ANOVA) for repeated measures to test for within—and between—group effects. The regression lines were computed using the least squares procedure; the slopes were compared; regressions were calculated using the peak pressure point reached for each maneuver; and at least three points of the descending part of the curve for each subject. We excluded the "gentle Valsalva" and the knee bend maneuvers since the measurement of the releasing part of curve was inaccurate.

RESULTS

Peak ITP Reached

ITP levels were significantly higher than the standard maximal isometric effort during maximal Valsalva maneuver ($136\% \pm 11$, $p < 0.05$), cough ($133\% \pm 7$, $p < 0.05$), and breath-hold knee bend ($172\% \pm 14$, $p < 0.001$). Free knee bend ITP levels were similar to the standard isometric effort ($92\% \pm 14$, $p > 0.05$) whereas "Divers' Valsalva maneuver" (i.e., "gentle" Valsalva) produced ITPs significantly lower than the standard ($25\% \pm 6$, $p < 0,001$).

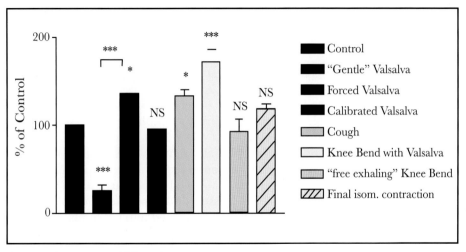

Figure 1. Comparison of ITP peaks
   NS: >0.05; *: p <0.05; ***: p <0.001
   Difference between "gentle Valsalva" and Forced Valsalva: ***

Slope of ITP Curves

Regression analysis yielded no statistical difference between the downward slopes of the various maneuvers ($p = 0.1447$). Accordingly, all the regression lines could be pooled into a single line with a common slope of -3.17. Thus, independent of the initial ITP peak or the duration of the maneuver, release of ITP followed a similar decay line. However, this does not imply that the maneuvers had similar cardiovascular effects.

Much emphasis has been placed on using coughing as a screening technique for intracardiac shunts. Even though the pressure excursion may be comparable to the other maneuvers, the effect on peripheral blood pooling is not the same; significant blood pooling is required for effective opening of a *foramen ovale* after releasing ITP (Siostrzonek et al., 1991).

DISCUSSION

The Valsalva maneuver is used commonly to augment contrast echocardiography sensitivity. Typically, it consists of a manual blockage of the nostrils, followed by a forced expiration against closed mouth and nose, to provoke an augmentation of the pressure in the nasopharyngeal cavity. Inevitably, this maneuver provokes a rise in intrathoracic pressure.

There are six major components during a Valsalva maneuver (Germonpre et al., 1998b): the initial inhalation phase, exhalation phase, straining phase, releasing phase and finally a second inhalation and exhalation phase (Cambier et al., 1993). Each phase is accompanied by changes in airway and intrathoracic pressure. These pressure changes interfere with the right and left atrial pressure curves.

During the initial inhalation phase, there is an increase in intrathoracic pressure resulting in a greater right atrial pressure relative to the left and an increased gradient between the extrathoracic veins and the right atrium. This generates an influx of blood from the superior and inferior vena cava with right atrial filling. This, combined with the increased filling capacity of the expanded lungs, causes a subsequent decrease in left atrial return and pressure.

During the exhaling phase against resistance, the airway and intrathoracic pressures increase with consequent left atrial pressure predominance. The increased intrathoracic pressure reduces the systemic venous return to the heart. Initially, the back pressure results in distention of peripheral veins up to the limits of available venous capacity. This occurs at the expense of flow through the central veins and explains the drop in right ventricular stroke volume (Versprille et al., 1982). During the first few heartbeats following the release of the Valsalva maneuver, Lee and co-workers (Lee et al., 1954; Cambier et al., 1990) observed an increase in right atrial pressure above the level of the pulmonary wedge pressure and therefore, presumably, also above the left atrial pressure. Other maneuvers that lead to similar increases in ITP might therefore be expected to have similar results.

From our investigations, we have shown that the usual Valsalva maneuver, as used by divers to equalize the pressure in their middle ear cavities, only causes a very slight rise in ITP and this is usually only of very short duration. It is therefore unlikely to induce major blood shifts or the pressure changes that might open a PFO. On the other hand, if the Valsalva maneuver is "forced," these changes may well occur ($p < 0.001$). Here the rise of ITP is even greater than that which is obtained by maximal isometric effort.

Embolization has been reported in patients with PFO during Valsalva maneuver (Lee et al., 1954). Based on this and other PFO studies (Moon et al., 1989; Rohr Lefloch, 1994), it has become common to advise divers with PFOs not to perform any Valsalva maneuvers during or after ascent from their dives (e.g., to lift heavy objects or to relieve residual pressure differences in the middle ears using Valsalva maneuvers). The reason for the recommendation is that silent bubbles can be present in the central venous blood for up to two hours after a deep dive (Wilmshurst et al., 1989). Our results suggest this only applies to forced Valsalva maneuvers. Indeed, divers should be taught to avoid forceful Valsalva maneuvers to equalize middle ear pressures; they should avoid using their abdominal muscles as the intra-abdominal pressure can also interfere with ITP (Eckenhoff et al., 1990). Only jaw and throat muscles should be used and this should receive special attention during dive training (Cresswell et al., 1992). In addition the recommendation should be extended towards avoiding sustained isometric exercise or abdominal strains (e.g., lifting of heavy equipment and dive tanks; orally inflating buoyancy control device at the surface; and even defecation).

The anatomical characteristics of PFO are well known (Cambier, 1993). The repeated rebound blood shift and subsequent rise in right atrial pressure may eventually even open previously closed, but only lightly fused, *Foramina Ovale*; a minimally patent Foramen Ovale may even increase in size over time. This hypothesis, yet unproven, is circumstantially supported by two findings. Firstly, anatomical studies indicate that, in older age groups, the incidence of PFO is lower, but the average diameter is larger. Secondly, from our own experience, several older and experienced divers have been struck by repeated episodes of "unexplained DCI" (i.e. without having violated currently accepted diving technical rules, considered as "safe") after having performed sometimes more than 1000 dives without any problem. In all of these divers, a large PFO was detected on c-TEE.

TABLE 2. INTRATHORACIC PRESSURE PEAK VALUE FOR VARIOUS MANEUVERS

Maneuver	Percentage (%)	Δ Pressure (mm H$_g$)
Control	100	78±5
Ear Equalizing Maneuver	25±6	19.5±4.7
Forced Equalizing Valsalva	136±11	106.1±8.6
Free Exhaling Knee Bend	92±14	71.8±11
Breath-Hold Knee Bend	172±14	134.2±11
Cough	133±7	103.7±5.5

Intrathoracic mean pressure values (n=16)

CONCLUSIONS

With the exception of minimal pressure Valsalva maneuvers, any prolonged and forced straining maneuver is prone to cause post-release, central blood shifts due to a combination of the high ITP and greater "pooling" of blood. (Table 2).

Even though the mechanisms for raising and lowering ITP may be different for these various maneuvers, the ITP release curves are identical (i.e., the slopes of the regression lines are the same). Therefore, divers (particularly those with confirmed PFOs) should avoid all maneuvers or forms of exercise that are likely to cause a prolonged rise in ITP after diving. This is of particular importance for a period of approximately two hours after diving when significant quantities of venous gas emboli may be present. Strenuous arm and leg exercises (such as SCUBA gear tank handling and boarding the dive boat with full equipment) should also be avoided after deep and decompression dives.

Even though a PFO may certainly permit embolization of nitrogen bubbles, it is *the bubbles* rather than the PFO that are the actual problem. Accordingly, if venous gas bubbles can be eliminated, the presence of intra-cardiac or even trans-pulmonary shunts becomes irrelevant. Several simple measures can significantly reduce the quantity of nitrogen bubbles after a dive. These are discussed in more detail in another chapter. They include not diving deeper than 30m; ascending at a rate not significantly faster *or slower* than 10m/minute; performing empirical deep and shallow "safety stops" of 3–5 minutes on no-decompression dives greater than 25 msw (82 fsw) meters. These measures have all been shown to substantially reduce venous nitrogen bubble loads after a dive (Wilmshurst et al., 1989; Marroni et al., 2004a).

SOME HYPOBARIC CONSIDERATIONS

Although altitude and diving-related dysbaric illnesses are closely related, the differences are of particular interest. Divers enter an environment of increased pressure after which they decompress. Astronauts face decompression situations from their baseline pressurized environment, such as with Extravehicular Activity (EVA). In addition, divers perform their duties or activities while under pressure after which they decompress. Astronauts perform their functions during a state of decompression after which they return to pressure (Waligora et al., 1987; Waligora et al., 1991). Divers working in saturation environments are decompressed slowly to allow them to desaturate almost completely by the time they reach the surface. This is impractical for astronauts. They therefore perform oxygen prebreathing, with or without exercise, to hasten the denitrogenation allowing them to decompress more quickly.

As far as PFO is concerned, astronauts—unlike divers—fortunately do not experience prolonged increases in intrathoracic pressure, unless they happen to manipulate heavy objects or experience significant exertion in space (Balestra et al., 1998). Oxygen prebreathing schedules also significantly reduce DCI risk (Horrigan et al. 1989). Even if venous gas bubbles were to arterialize, they would embolize tissue beds that were not significantly saturated with inert gas. Consequently, they would be less likely to grow. The converse situation would occur in divers—as described by the well-known Hennessy model of arterial bubbles (Hennessy and Hempleman, 1977) (Figure 2).

This model delineates the consequences of cavitation bubbles entering the circulatory system in a saturated state. This also partially applies to hypobaric situations where such cavitations are augmented. On the other hand, saturation and tribonucleation are reduced in these environments (Garret, 1990).

Once again, this illustrates that the causes for DCI are multifactorial; PFO is only one of many possibilities. Circulating bubbles from micro embolization may be of even greater importance (Balestra, 2000).

Positive Pressure Breathing (PPB) used during altitude flights may impose DCI risks on individuals with PFO (Garret, 1990). There have been

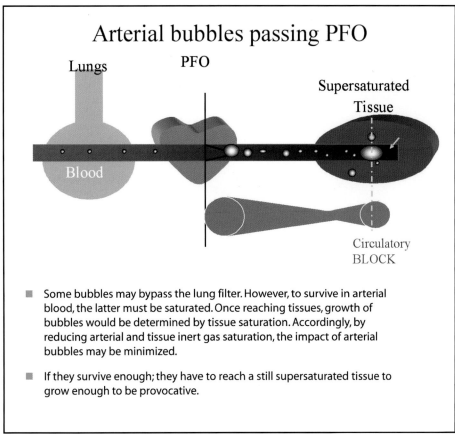

Figure 2. Hennessy's model for provocative arterial bubbles.

conflicting reports as to whether positive pressure (PEEP) breathing does (Cujec et al., 1993) or does not provoke (Zasslow et al., 1988) a reversal of interatrial pressures. Proponents of this hypothesis suggest that PEEP breathing has similar effects as PPB.

NOTES

CHAPTER 8

PFO DETECTION IN DIVERS—METHODOLOGICAL ASPECTS

INTRODUCTION

Recent publications have emphasized the importance of standardizing c-TEE. Although most agree that the technique is relatively benign (Fisher, et al., 1995), there is no consensus on quantifying and evaluating the results.

Mas, et al. used semi quantitative c-TEE to determine the size of patency of the Foramen Ovale (PFO) in their patient groups (Mas, et al., 2001). They stated that there was a substantial degree of disagreement amongst the three reviewers of the c-TEE video recordings. Others have also studied the variability in PFO detection and have shown significant discrepancies (Fisher, et al., 1995; Nygren and Jogestrand, 1998; Greim, et al., 2001; Ha, et al., 2001; Kampen, et al., 2001; Pfleger, et al., 2001; Cabanes, et al., 2002).

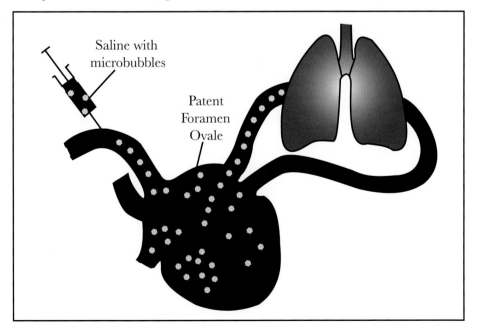

Figure 1. Schematic view of the contrast injection during TEE examination.

Schuchlenz, et al. (Schuchlenz, et al., 2002a) have confirmed that the degree of shunting of contrast solution injected into an antecubital vein is inferior to injections into the femoral vein; an observation previously made by Gin, et al. nine years earlier (Gin, et al., 1993); and by Hamann, et al. four years earlier (Hamann, et al., 1998). However this lack of consistency is probably due to the absence of an effective straining maneuver able to redirect flow of contrast through a PFO after entering from the superior vena cava rather than relying on preferential flow from the Inferior Caval Vein (ICV) towards the fossa ovalis (Rouvière and Delmas, 1985). It is striking that none of the studies offer a precise description of the nature and duration of the straining maneuver—a serious methodological flaw in our view.

PROPOSAL

We have observed that, to achieve adequate contrast mixing in the right atrium, the duration of the straining maneuver is more important than the actual intrathoracic pressure obtained (Balestra, et al., 1998). Based on this observation, we proposed a standardized straining maneuver for c-TEE examinations for PFO (Germonpre, et al., 1998b). The protocol is summarized below.

PROTOCOL

The following steps should provide greater consistency in evaluating PFO using c-TEE:

1. Identify the interatrial septum in long-axis view, focusing on the separation plane between septum primum and secundum (Schuchlenz, et al., 2000)
2. Perform an initial straining maneuver in order to exclude false respiratory contrast (Van Camp, et al., 1994)
3. Perform a first contrast study, using the same straining maneuver:

   - After a medium to deep inspiration, and with closed glottis, perform an abdominal pressure increase ("push down in the abdomen") while the investigator counts slowly to 10.
   - Keep the TEE probe immobile, even if the heart seems to shift slightly from view during this maneuver.
   - Inject contrast medium (in our case, agitated saline 9.5ml + 0.5ml air) through a large-bore catheter in an elbow vein, after 7–8 seconds of straining.
   - When the first contrast bubbles appear in the right atrium, instruct the patient to exhale normally.
   - Observe and grade right-to-left shunting of contrast bubbles within the first three heartbeats after release of the straining maneuver: Grade 0–no passage; Grade I–less than 20 bubbles; and Grade II–more than 20 bubbles.

CONCLUSIONS

Using this standardised straining maneuver, we have been able to show a high level of correlation between Grade II PFO and cerebral DCI in sports divers. The hypothesis is paradoxical embolization of nitrogen bubbles arising predominantly from the lower extremities and reaching the heart via the inferior vena cava—a mechanism similar to that proposed for unexplained stroke (Van Camp, et al., 1993).

The use of spontaneous shunting (i.e., without straining maneuver) due to the post-embryological anatomy and flow characteristics, is unnecessary and not appropriate. However, in patients incapable of performing a proper straining maneuver, injection of contrast should rather be performed through the femoral vein.

Using this above-mentioned technique, we were able to detect reliably, reproducibly and unequivocally the presence of PFO with grading as described above. A simple check of the proper contrast injection can be done by observing a full opacification of the right atrium, with contrast filling up to the septum (Balestra, et al., 2002).

In the following chapter, we introduce the hypothesis, formulated in 1998, that the pevalence of PFO seemed to change in a group of dives during follow-up over several years and that this appeared to be higher than the prevalence in the normal population.

NOTES

CHAPTER 9

TIME RELATED OPENING OF THE FORAMEN OVALE IN DIVERS

The presence of a PFO has been associated with a higher incidence of neurological DCI in SCUBA divers. Using a highly standardized semi-quantified c-TEE, we tested and re-tested a group of 33 divers after an interval of seven years. We found that 12% (n=4) of the tested divers had experienced an increased in the size of the PFO, and that in a further 12% (n=4) a PFO was found where previously there was none. We hypothesized that, in the course of adult life, PFO's may increase in size or even appear "de novo."

METHODS

A group of 33 divers who had undergone previous investigation for PFO (using a strictly standardized c-TEE technique in the period 1994–1996) gave their informed consent for re-evaluation using the same technique, 6–8 years later. The group consisted of 33 divers of whom 15 had suffered DCI previously, and 16 who never had DCI but had served as matched controls for the study. All divers had continued diving; none had not suffered DCI since their first c-TEE.

PFO assessment involved echocardiographic visualization of the inter-atrial septum via TEE, whereafter 10cc agitated saline was injected into an antecubital vein while the subjects performed a prolonged straining maneuver (i.e., a modified Valsalva strain for at least ten seconds) (Balestra et al., 1998)). Upon arrival of contrast in the right atrium, the subject was instructed to release the straining and breathe normally. Contrast passage into the left atrium within three cardiac cycles was considered proof of paradoxical embolism through a PFO. A test was considered negative if, after three attempts, no contrast passage was observed while the right atrium was completely filled with contrast. In order to exclude "false respiratory contrast," a straining maneuver and release was performed before the first contrast injection (Germonpre et al., 1998b).

PFO was semi-quantified according to the degree of paradoxical contrast passage (Grade 0: no bubble passage; Grade I: <20 bubbles; Grade II: > 20 bubbles).

RESULTS

The initial prevalence of PFO in this group of divers was 42.5% (14/33), of whom five (36%) had a Grade I and nine (64%) had a Grade II PFO. The mean years of diving between the two c-TEE assessments was 7.28 and the mean number of dives was 283 (39 dives/year). The prevalence of PFO during the second assessment was 51.5% (17/33).

Of the 19 divers who initially presented without a PFO, three were found to have a Grade I PFO after a mean of 7.6 years and 556 dives. One diver had a Grade II PFO (after seven years, 150 dives). Fifteen divers were still classified Grade 0 (mean 7.36 years; 292 dives).

Of the five divers with an initial Grade I PFO, four were found to have a Grade II PFO (mean 7.75 years; 225 dives). One diver with a former PFO was found to be contrast negative (seven years; 100 dives).

TABLE 1. PFO IN DIVERS: RESULTS

	Changed	Unchanged
No PFO	4	15
PFO 1	5	0
PFO 2	0	9

DISCUSSION

Autopsy assessment of 965 heart specimens has suggested that the prevalence of PFO decreases, while the mean size of the remaining PFO's increases with age (Hagen et al., 1984). This is consistent with our findings in which—after seven years—four divers had an increase in PFO's classification from Grade I to Grade II, while one diver's Grade I PFO spontaneously closed. However, it was a novel discovery that four divers presented with PFO whereas seven years before they had been contrast negative.

Mechanisms for de novo opening of PFO's could involve diving-related phenomena, such as variations in the right atrial pressures during the end-stages of, or events immediately following, a dive. However, such pressure fluctuations are equally associated with straining-release events associated with certain types of exercise and activities of daily living. Accordingly, no specific diving-related hypothesis is suggested at this time.

We consider the de novo opening of four PFO's an important finding because this may suggest that divers may develop greater susceptibility for neurological DCI over time (Germonpre, 2005; Germonpre et al., 2005).

Another hypothesis is that these divers had minute PFO's at the initial examination, allowing no bubble passage at all, and that they became Grade I (permeable) over the course of these seven years. We could thus hypothesise a continuum of increasing permeability, where gradually more and more bubbles can be shunted through the interatrial septum. If this hypothesis were true, older divers would possibly be at increased risk for cerebral DCI, whether clinically overt or not.

The effects of repetitive nitrogen bubble embolization of the brain have worried researchers for years. Although unlikely after mild dive profiles, as described by the Hennessy model (see 'Some Hypobaric Considerations' in the chapter entitled "Intrathoracic Pressure Changes After Valsalva Strain and Other Manuevers"), embolization following dives with greater tissue saturations may have more serious consequences.

NOTES

CHAPTER 10

BRAIN MAGNETIC RESONANCE IMAGING (MRI) HYPERINTENSE SPOTS IN DIVERS

INTRODUCTION

Given the very sensitive nature of brain tissue, there is potential cause for concern about the long-term effects of scuba diving and neurological DCI. To date, however, no consensus exists whether diving per se causes brain damage or not—as emphasized in recent literature (Wilmshurst, 1997). However, the uncertainty remains and one is left with the distinct impression that professional diving may indeed cause brain damage and neuropsychological impairment, irrespective of whether episodes of DCI were recorded or treated (Calder, et al., 1987; Palmer, et al., 1987; Rinck, et al., 1991; Dujic, et al., 1993). Similar concerns exist for sport scuba diving although it has been afforded little attention.

Neurological Long-Term Effects of Professional Diving

Todnem, et al. reported that long-term neurological findings were correlated highly significantly with exposure to deep professional diving. However the abnormal magnetic resonance imaging (MRI)[†] findings did not offer a specific explanation (Todnem, et al., 1991). Nevertheless, even if abnormal MRI findings have not yet been conclusively associated with DCI there still appear to be changes in the brain associated with professional scuba diving.

Fueredi, et al. have shown that the risk for white-matter injury is greater in compressed air workers than age- and occupationally-matched, non-diving, control subjects (Fueredi, et al., 1991).

Yanagawa, et al. observed larger number of abnormalities on MRI (n=9) in a cohort of 25 Coast Guard scuba divers than in a matched control group

---

† Magnetic resonance imaging is a method used to visualize parts of the human body without the need for radio activity (e.g., x-rays or CT scanning). It employs a powerful magnetic field to change the orientation of hydrogen atom predominately in water molecules in the body in such a way that they subsequently spin back and release radiowaves. These can then be read by a specialized receiver and be used to generate images. Depending on the way in which the magnetism is employed and the way in which the hydrogen atoms 'relax" a distinction can be made between free water and bound (tissue or intercellular) water, and even other compounds. The method thereby allows distinction between blood, inflammation, edema (swelling), tissue death necrosis, bruising (contusion), etc.

(n=2) (Yanagawa, et al., 1998), supporting previous works (Rinck, et al., 1991; Reuter, et al., 1997; Sparacia, et al., 1997).

In support of these concerns, some studies using neuropsychological testing have indeed shown permanent memory impairment and depression related to professional diving activity (Aarli, et al., 1985; Rinck, et al., 1991; Di Piero, et al., 2002).

Then again, others have yielded negative results. Cordes, et al. study examined 24 professional divers without any DCI history using radiologic and neuropsychologic tests and compared the results to a control group of 24 non-diving healthy volunteers (Cordes, et al., 2000). The investigators found that six divers (25%) had unidentified bright objects on MRI (UBO's), whereas the control group had ten individuals with UBO's (42%). Accordingly, no statistical difference was found between the divers and the control group when comparing the number and the size of the UBO's, nor was there statistical difference in their psychometric evaluations.

Neurological Long-Term Effects of Sport Scuba Diving

In a well known paper, Reul, et al. stressed the risk of accumulating lesions in the central nervous system as a result of diving (Reul, et al., 1995). In their research, they found significantly more hyperintense signals in the brain and spinal cord of amateur divers compared to age- and gender-matched non-diving controls. Therefore, they suggested that permanent neuropsychological changes may be present and could be the result of sub-clinical intravascular gas bubbles. These observations have contributed to the ongoing debate regarding the safety of recreational diving. Could repeated showers of venous gas bubbles be causing permanent damage, especially to the central nervous system? Before answering the question from the conclusions of Reul's study, certain issues should be raised about the way the study was performed. For instance, there are concerns about the selection of their subjects; unknown reproducibility of MRI interpretation; incomplete assessment of possible confounding factors (e.g., risk factors for cerebral vascular disease); and lack of longitudinal follow-up and neuropsychological evaluation. The authors attributed any lesions found in the brain (cortical gray matter, subcortical white matter, central white matter, basal ganglia, cerebellum, brain stem or central white matter) to diving and classified them by number and size. However the sensitivity and specificity of their findings were not validated and misinterpretation cannot be excluded (Jungreis, et al., 1988; Heier, et al., 1989).

Nevertheless, the issue of scuba diving vs. brain damage remains a critical one that has yet to be solved (Palmer, et al., 1992). To our knowledge, there are very few uncontrolled studies on neurological dysfunction or neuropsychological impairment due to recreational or sport diving (Edmonds and Boughton, 1985; Tetzlaff, et al., 1999). The discussion therefore continues (Hovens, et al., 1995; Rogers, 1995; Wilmshurst, et al., 1995).

The current situation has been succinctly summarized as follows by Wilmshurst in an editorial of the British Medical Journal (Wilmshurst, 1997):

    a. There is no consensus regarding brain damage caused exclusively by diving;

    b. There are no adequate data supporting that diving per se causes cerebral functional abnormalities;

c. MRI examination provides non-specific information and does not
always reveal abnormalities in cases of clear neurological DCI; and

d. MRI findings do not correlate with the results of psychometric tests
or electroencephalograms.

The possibility of visualizing lesions by newer MRI techniques is
intriguing as it may assist in unraveling the relevance to diving (Todnem,
et al., 1991; Tetzlaff, et al., 1999). These include diffusion and perfusion-
weighted imaging and FLAIR (Fluid Attenuated Inversion Recovery).

Although the question whether SCUBA diving by itself can cause brain
damage remains unanswered, it has been known for a long time that DCI
certainly can cause permanent neurological damage. Yet, even here, evidence has been conflicting. Kelleher, et al. reviewed 214 cases of neurological DCI and noticed that the type and extent of initial symptoms
determined ultimate recovery (Kelleher, et al., 1996). Murrison, et al. on
the other hand found no evidence for persistent neurological damage after
full clinical recovery at 17 months follow-up of a cohort of 40 commercial
divers (McQueen, et al., 1994). Some authors have correlated these findings to the presence of PFO. Knauth and collaborators (Knauth, et al., 1997)
analyzed 87 experienced divers (average of 500 logged dives) without overt or
disclosed DCI episodes. They discovered that there was an increased prevalence of multiple brain lesions in a small subgroup of divers without a history
of "Type 2" DCI (DCI). They concluded that these lesions were the consequence of subclinical gas embolism through a Patent Foramen Ovale (PFO).
However, several important remarks have to be made that considerably weak-
en these conclusions.

Firstly, the authors stated that, unlike the Reul study (Reul, et al.,
1995), self-selection bias was not a problem—subjects were not aware of
having PFO or not. However there is a flaw in this reasoning: by soliciting
divers to participate in a study examining possible brain damage from
SCUBA diving one may still self-select divers who experienced previous
minor symptoms—irrespective of whether the diagnosis of DCI was ever
made (Germonpré, et al., 1996).

Secondly, the authors performed transcranial Doppler after bubble
contrast injection which, unfortunately, contained some questionable
methodological aspects in terms of contrast production and straining procedures. Their results were as follows:

- Seven out of 62 divers without PFO had Unidentified Bright
  Objects (UBO's—one each); and
- Four out of 25 divers with a PFO had UBO's. Among them, one
  with a small PFO had only a single UBO whereas the other three
  had 80% of the total number of UBO's (41).

Although this difference was statistically significant, it had very low
power. If only one of the three divers with multiple brain lesions was
excluded from the study, statistical significance would not have been
reached (p=0.075 instead of 0.022).

Thirdly, although transcranial Doppler measurements accurately detected
right-to-left shunts, they would not be able to differentiate between PFO and

other arteriovenous shunts, such as Atrial Septal Defects and pulmonary shunts. Since these abnormalities were not specifically excluded in the subjects, it is, in our view, inappropriate to conclude that paradoxical embolism necessarily occurred via a PFO.

Another recent Swiss study (Schwerzmann and Seiler, 2001) studied the brain MRI images of 52 non-professional divers and performed c-TEE on them for the presence of a PFO. They then compared the incidence of UBO and PFO with a control group of 52 non-diving volunteers. The authors concluded that there was a greater prevalence of UBO's in divers with PFO—similar to the findings of others (Reul et al., 1995; Knauth et al., 1997))—but added that the UBO prevalence was still greater in divers without PFO's than in non-diving controls. They therefore concluded that the "lesions" were of vascular origin; that PFO was the causal reason for the presumed paradoxical embolizations; and that diving *per se* was therefore a dangerous activity for the central nervous tissue. Even if these findings were true, the impact of safer diving techniques needs to be considered, irrespective of the presence of PFO, before making a generalized statement about the safety of recreational diving.

Many questions remain to be answered, and the methodologies of these various studies remain troublesome. Accordingly, we decided to perform a study of our own to answer some of the provocative questions and to address specifically the problems with standardization as well as confounding risk factors related to cerebral vascular disease vs. PFO.

METHODS

Population

The experimental group consisted of 54 divers who were randomly chosen among a group of 120. The control group was composed of 34 non-diving healthy volunteers age 23–37 (26 +/- 3.5 years). The total time required for the study was two years and inevitably some selected subjects left the study before completing all the tests. Forty-two divers finished the study protocol (age: 36 +/- 4.8). The overall characteristics of the study population (inclusion and exclusion criteria) were as follows:

- RECREATIONAL DIVERS: as diving procedures and breathing gases differ between recreational and professional divers, conclusions that apply to the one group do not necessarily apply to the other. This was a study on recreational diving.
- AGE LESS THAN 41: the incidence of asymptomatic UBO's or hyperintense spots increases beyond age 50; we therefore limited the inclusion criterion to 40 years (Thompson-Schill et al., 2002; Taylor et al., 2003)
- SIGNIFICANT NUMBER OF LOGGED DIVES: we included only divers with at least 200 logged dives. In previous studies authors had collated the results of divers with between 40 and 2000 dives (Reul et al., 1995; Knauth et al., 1997; Schwerzmann and Seiler, 2001). If UBO's are related to the diving practice, then the number of dives should be considered as an inclusion criterion.

- NO HISTORY OF DCI: DCI manifestations are usually evident; nevertheless, some subclinical DCI and particularly some transient cerebral vascular bubbles could present as minor, passing episodes of dizziness, rather than "true" DCI. If this factor is not taken into account, it is possible that "worried" divers—who had felt "something" but did not want to be labeled as having suffered DCI—could present themselves as candidates for the study for their own peace of mind. This could introduce bias. Accordingly, we performed randomization of the volunteers (one in three, according to a computer-generated random number list).

Data Collection

Questionnaire

Every participant, after being fully informed and signing the informed consent document, filled in a complete medical questionnaire:

- Personal information
- Data concerning dive experience: level of certification; number of dives to date; average depth; maximum depth; breathing mixture used; equalizing technique used, etc.
- Physical condition: subjective evaluation of the individual's own physical condition.
- Medical history

Magnetic resonance imaging

All the exams were performed on a 1.5 Tesla machine. The slices were 5 mm thickness (standard brain examination) in the following three planes: axial, sagittal, and frontal. Three different sequences were used: Sagittal T1; Axial T2; Axial FLAIR.

The tissues with a long relaxation time on MRI, like CSF or the vascular bed, appear more intense (hypersignal) on T2 sequence.

By choosing a different relaxation time, liquid spaces can be shown—T1 sequence. Ischemic zones can then be detected by comparing the two sequences. In doing so possible ambiguities between ischemic zones and liquid spaces can be avoided. Finally, a UBO is definitively identified only if it appears clearly in T2 and FLAIR on the same slice.

The images were independently evaluated by two neuroradiologists, and if there was disagreement, a third one was consulted. After identification of the UBO's, their number, size and anatomical location were recorded. Other visible pathologies or peculiarities (sinusitis, cysts, etc.) were also recorded.

Transesophageal echocardiography (c-TEE)

Finally, the participants underwent standardized c-TEE as previously described. The protocol made provision for analysis of the recorded images by an independent cardiologist. These included:

- Mobility of the interatrial septum (mm) or aneurism;
- Distal (valvular) part of the septum (sealed or unsealed);
- Right-to-left contrast passage during spontaneous respiration (with semi quantification of bubble passage); and

- Right-to-left contrast passage after straining manoeuvre (with semi-quantification of bubble passage).

ANALYSIS
Demographics

The control group consisted of young, healthy students of the Institute for Physical Education. The controls were somewhat younger than the divers and included more smokers, but we accepted the difference for the following reasons:

- Current medical literature suggests that asymptomatic cerebral white matter spots (UBO's) are not anticipated in the general population below 40 years (Lechner et al., 1988; Bryan et al., 1999; Ding et al., 2003). As both groups fell within this range, the slight differences were not considered clinically important;
- Although there is a weak correlation (r=0.16) between smoking and UBO's in older patient groups, as recorded in 253 patients by Fukuda et al (Fukuda and Kitani, 1996), this has not been demonstrated in young adults (Yamashita et al., 1996). Moreover, if there were to be a difference, it would be higher in the control group (see "Discussion" below); and
- Recreational drug use was recorded as part of the questionnaire; frequent or habitual use was considered an exclusion criterion (Bartzokis et al., 1999a; Bartzokis et al., 1999b; O'Leary et al., 2002).

MRI Data

TABLE 1. POPULATION CHARACTERISTICS FOR THE BRAIN MRI STUDY

POPULATION CHARATERISTICS	DIVERS	NON DIVERS
Age (yrs) (mean+/−SD)	36 ± 4.9	26.3 ± 3.5
Males (%)	91%	50%
Regular alcohol consumption, n (%)	9(23)	11(33)
Regular Smoking, n (%)	3(7)	23(67)
Presence of UBO, n (%)	5(12)	3(9)
Area (mm) of UBO's (mean +/−SD)	4.8 ± 2.8	1.33 ± 0.6

The MRI analysis showed that five out of the 42 divers (12%) had one UBO's each (i.e., five UBO's), their sizes varied from 2–10 mm². Two UBO's were located in the right frontal area; one in the right temporal area; one in the posterior parietal space; and one in the left frontal area. Two divers presented with a diffuse lacunar syndrome and were excluded because this was attributed to subclinical Multiple Sclerosis (exclusion criterion). In the non-diving population, three of the 34 participants (9%)

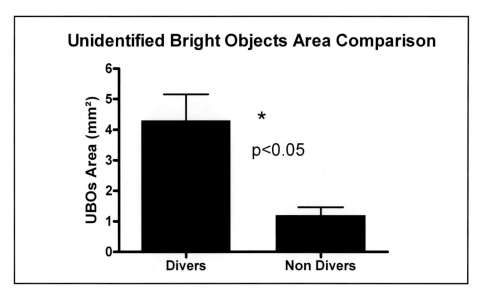

Figure 1. Comparison of UBO size between divers and controls.

had UBO's ranging from 1–2 mm^2: one had an isolated UBO and two
had multifocal UBO's. One non-diver was excluded due to the diagnosis
of multiple sclerosis. All participants with suspected multiple sclerosis
were sent to a neurologist for appropriate management.

For the purpose of internal control, three subjects (one control; two
divers) agreed to undergo a second MRI examination some time afterwards
(up to one year). The second examination was entirely consistent with the first.

Although the number of UBO's was greater in divers than the controls
(7% vs. 4%), this did not reach statistical significance (Fisher's Exact Test;

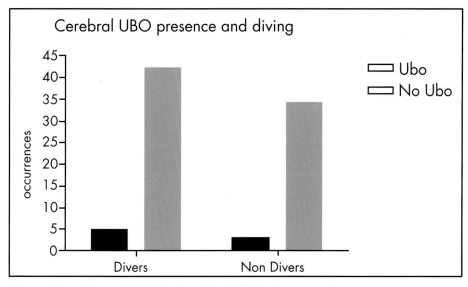

Figure 2. Prevalence of UBO's in divers (no DCI history) and non-divers

TABLE 2. PRESENCE AND GRADING OF PFO IN THE DIVERS STUDIED

Divers without PFO		15/42	35.7%
Divers with PFO		**27/42**	**64.3%**
PFO: Grades I and II (n=27)	Grade I	11/27	40.7%
	Grade II	16/27	59.3%
PFO: All Grades (n=42)	Grade 0	15/42	35.7%
	Grade I	11/42	26.2%
	Grade II	16/42	38.1%

p=0.72). No statistical difference was found when comparing the divers to non-divers with multifocal UBO's (p=0.11).

However, there was a statistical difference in the size (area) of the UBO's between the two groups (p=0.04).

Transesophageal Echocardiography

Using the gold standard to detect PFO (c-TEE) we found a larger than expected proportion of PFO's in the diving population (64.3%); autopsy data for this age group is between 20% and 25% (Hagen et al., 1984).

The relatively high number of Grade II PFO's amongst the experienced divers is unusual. This may be consistent with our hypothesis that some experienced divers appear to develop increased patency over time.

Correlation Between c-TEE and MRI

In total five UBO's were detected in five out of 42 divers; two had a PFO and three did not (5% vs. 8% of the divers examined). This was not statistically significant and this negative finding is at odds with the conclusions proposed in earlier publications (Reul et al., 1995; Knauth et al., 1997; Hierholzer et al., 2000). On the other hand it is consistent with those of more recent studies (Cordes et al., 2000; Gerriets et al., 2000; Farkas et al., 2001). Given the presumed pathophysiological mechanism for ischemic brain spots i.e., paradoxical embolization of bubbles (Buttinelli et al., 2002) or thromboemboli (Schuchlenz et al., 2000; Schuchlenz et al., 2002a), the relationship between PFO and UBO's should have been stronger.

Even when PFO grade is related to the presence of UBO's, there is no statistical difference between any of the subgroups (p=0.95).

To analyze whether there was a trend between the UBO's and the size of the PFO's we performed a Chi-squared test for independence and trends.

Chi-squared Test for Independence: p=0.9522.

Row and column variables were not significantly associated.

Chi-Squared Test for Trend: p=0.8900.

No significant linear trend exists amongst the ordered categories.

If we associate the "All-PFO" Population versus "No PFO" according to a Fisher's Exact Test, no statistical evidence is found.

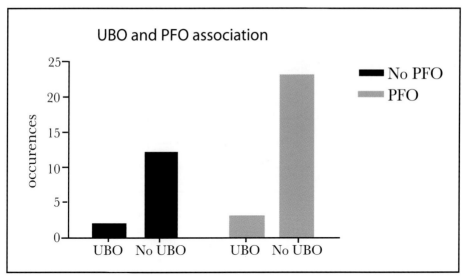

Figure 3. PFO vs. UBO—relative relationships.

TABLE 3. GRADING AND PRESENCE OF UBO'S (STATISTICAL ANALYSIS); P=0.95

	PFO Grade 0	PFO Grade I	PFO Grade II	Total
UBO	2 (5%)	1 (3%)	2 (5%)	5 (13%)
No UBO	12 (30%)	9 (22%)	14 (35%)	35 (87%)
Total	14 (35%)	10 (25%)	16 (40%)	40 (100%)

TABLE 4.

Column	Total	Percent
PFO 0	14	35.00%
PFO 1	10	25.00%
PFO 2	16	40.00%
Total	40	100.00%

TABLE 5.

	No PFO	PFO	Total
UBO	2	3	5
	(5%)	(8%)	(13%)
No UBO	12	23	35
	(30%)	(57%)	(88%)
Total	14	26	40
	(35%)	(65%)	(100%)

Again, our results differ from those previously reported by some (Schuchlenz et al., 2000; Schuchlenz et al., 2002b) but are consistent with others (Cordes et al., 2000; Gerriets et al., 2000).

Diving Population Characteristics

To determine the possibility of UBO's being attributable to other diving-related risk factors or specific diving habits, all participants completed a detailed questionnaire that yielded the following results:

Medical risk factors for UBO's such as migraine, hypertension, surgi-

TABLE 6. DIVING HABITS AND CORRELATION WITH UBO'S PRESENCE AND SIZE

DIVING PROFILE	UBO PRESENCE	SIZE OF UBO'S
Total N° of Dives	r = 0.16	r = 0.20
Equalizing ears technique	r = 0.12	r =0.12
Mean duration of dives	r = 0.27	r = 0.31
Diving depth > 40 m	r = 0.33	r = 0.08
No Deco limit dives	r = 0.36	r = 0.34
Respect of Safety stops	r = 0.31	r = 0.26

cal procedures, regular alcohol consumption, and smoking were examined but these failed to achieve statistical significance using Fisher's test. It was also confirmed that the mean age difference between the control group and the divers did not skew the results. As anticipated, no significant correlation was found between age and UBO's (r=0.11).

Specific Questions Related to PFO

In an effort to identify factors possibly inducing patency of foramen ovale (as detailed in the chapter entitled, "Time Related Opening of the Foramen Ovale in Divers"), a questionnaire was distributed to examine diving habits as well as other potential causes of prolonged, increased intrathoracic pressure (ITP) or increased right atrial pressure (IRAP).

Increases in IRAP have been observed during decompression; the mean pressure in the inferior vena cava was increased in a study of pigs (Vik et al., 1992, 1993), but then many down-to-earth human activities also raise ITP. For instance, individuals performing any exertion while maintaining a closed glottis or those playing wood-wind or brass musical instruments increase their intrathoracic pressure significantly (Balestra et al., 1998).

In summary:

- No significant correlation was found between age and PFO (r=0.18);
- No significant correlation was found between PFO and medical risk factors: migraine, hypertension, surgical interventions, regular alcohol consumption, and smoking; and
- No correlation was found between PFO Grade and increased intrathoracic pressure (e.g., exertion or relevant musical instruments) (r=0.26) or age (r=0.16).

TABLE 7. DIVE PROFILE AND PFO

DIVING PROFILE	UBO PRESENCE
Total N° of Dives	r = 0.003
Equalizing ears technique	r = 0.11
Mean duration of dives	r = 0.33
Diving depth > 40 m	r = 0.15
No Deco limit dives	r = 0.02

DISCUSSION

Some authors have reported an increased incidence of UBO's in recreational divers when compared to non diving populations (Reul et al., 1995; Knauth et al., 1997; Tetzlaff et al., 1999; Schwerzmann and Seiler, 2001; Buttinelli et al., 2002). Others have included divers who have experienced decompression illness (Torti et al., 2004). However, to understand whether uneventful recreational diving produces MRI hyperintense signals within the cerebral white matter, we compared 42 randomized divers to a control group of 34 non-diving volunteers.

Our results have allowed us to address two hypotheses: Whether an association exists between uneventful diving and the prevalence of UBO's; and whether these UBO's are related to PFO.

The MRI analysis showed that 5/42 divers and 3/34 non-divers had UBO's. This did not achieve statistical significance. The only difference was the size of UBO's which were greater in the diving population.

No individual, medical or lifestyle characteristics correlated to the size or number of UBO's for either group. Similarly, no correlation was found between the number or size of UBO's and the different diving parameters (i.e., years of diving; number of dives; mean depth; number of decompression dives; etc.).

This study was therefore unable to confirm that diving had any deleterious effects as determined by the presence of UBO's on MRI assessment. The only positive finding was that the size of UBO's was larger in the diving group.

The hypothesis of silent paradoxical embolization being a cause for cerebral UBO's is not supported by the study. Whether or not the UBO's were attributable to a vascular injury would require histological evaluation—an impractical option. Alternatively fractal geometry analysis (Porter et al., 1991; Meisel, 1992; Rigaut et al., 1998) could be used to test if the spatial distribution of the UBO's resembled the spatial distribution of the cerebral arterial bed. This is considered in the chapter entitled, "The Fractal Approach as a Tool to Understand Asymptomatic Brain Hyperintense MRI Signals." The next section is devoted to determining whether or not UBO's affect neuropsychometric and higher cerebral functions.

CHAPTER 11

NEUROPSYCHOMETRIC EVALUATION OF DIVERS

INTRODUCTION

Several studies and reports have raised concerns that divers with a PFO may arterialise nitrogen bubbles and thereby suffer subclinical brain embolism, even in the absence of clinical manifestations. This may ultimately lead to detectable brain white matter lesions on magnetic resonance imaging (MRI) and an associated deterioration in neuropsychometric function (Reul et al., 1995; Knauth et al., 1997, Todnem et al., 1991; Wilmshurst, 1997; van Dijk et al., 2002; den Heijer et al., 2003; Vermeer et al., 2003).

The exact nature of these "lesions" has not been established as being post-embolic or vascular. Accordingly, they are labelled as "UBO's" ("Unidentified Bright Objects"). If the above-mentioned fears were realized, diving with a PFO could constitute a serious health hazard (Edmonds and Boughton, 1985). After all, diving is a relatively young sport so that long-term health effects may only become noticeable after 10–20 years (Rogers, 1995).

Follow-up studies on elderly patients with white-matter lesions suggests that there is a greater association with Alzheimer-type dementia and general cognitive decline in otherwise healthy people over 60 (Vermeer et al., 2003). However, most of the published studies on divers suffer from potentially serious methodological shortcomings, so that their conclusions need to be verified before being accepted as truth.

As outlined before in the chapter entitled "Brain MRI Hyperintense Spots in Divers," most of the MRI studies in divers contained potential methodological flaws because:

- By using only "standard" MRI weighing techniques, "normal" variants such as Wirchow-Robin spaces could have been classified "abnormal";
- Not correlating abnormal findings to abnormalities in psychometric function. For UBO's to be anything more than morphological anomalies a pathological process or functional impairment should also be recorded.

In order to respond to as many of these concerns as possible, our diver population was carefully selected and MRI scanning and c-TEE examinations were performed using standardized and comprehensive diagnostic protocols (see "Proposal" in *PFO Detection in Divers*). Furthermore, neuropsychometric testing was performed using a computerized testing battery (Neuroscreen, IDEWE, Belgium), specially developed for detection of neurotoxic symptoms in industry workers. This testing battery was chosen as it permits the following (Michiels, 1999):

- measurement of neurotoxic effects (hypothesizing that nitrogen is a neuro-toxic agent)
- accounting for differences in education and schooling
- calculation of a "personal" reference score for each of the test items, obviating the need for a matched control population.

In addition, the battery has undergone thorough validation and evaluation on 1700 volunteers of different backgrounds. This includes recent internal validation by the researchers by means of a group of 161 "normal" subjects, and an "exposed" group of 96 persons (regular professional contact with potentially neurotoxic solvents). The battery is fully automated and computerized and shows excellent reproducibility of the test results.

Measured parameters were as follows:

- short-term working memory (Digit-Span Backwards test),
- associative speed (Digit-Symbol Substitution test), and
- reaction speed and hand-eye coordination (Trail Making test).

The entire testing procedure took 45 minutes on average, including an education and exposure questionnaire with a vocabulary test to determine general linguistic ability and education.

Results were analyzed using Mann-Whitney U-test, Fischer exact test and linear regression, via a computer-based standard statistical package (GraphPad Prism).

The Neuroscreen Data

General information

As a part of the enrollment, each subject was required to complete a questionnaire that solicited basic personal information as well as the number of years of schooling and highest level of education. These "scores" were then used to calculate an "expected" performance level for each neuropsychometric test to which the individual would be compared subsequently.

TABLE 1. EDUCATION SCORES CALCULATED BY THE NEUROSCREEN PROGRAM

Primary School = 1
Secondary School 3 yrs = 2
Secondary School 6 yrs = 3
Bachelor Degree = 4
University Master Degree = 5

The total number of school years achieved (primary included).

Neurological Anamnesis

This part of the test was designed to identify or account for other factors that might interfere with neurological performance (see below). As for the "education level," these results were used by the program to determine the "normal" levels of performance for each of the test items.

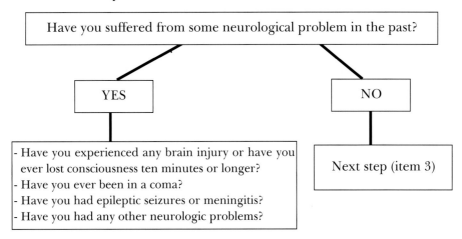

The "Simple Reaction Time" Test: (REA)

This test measured reaction time. The subjects were given a joystick to manipulate using the dominant hand. At the base of the joystick were located a blinking square red lamp (LED) and a push button. Whenever the red lamp turned on, the subject was required to push the button as quickly as possible. The red light signal appeared 60 times with a time interval between 2.5 and 5.5 seconds.

The software calculated:
- The mean reaction time (msec) (REA-gem)
- The stability of the reaction time (REA-stab)

The stability of the reaction time was calculated by using:
- A reaction time constant (REA-con).
- The standard deviation of the reaction time (REA-st-dev).
- The minimal reaction time (REA-min)

Data analysis permitted the evaluation of the time needed to process information in response to a simple stimulus (REA-gem); also some higher cerebral functions were required to keep the attention focused (REA-stab).

TABLE 2.

	Measure	**Evaluate**
(REA-gem)	Mean reaction time	Time to process information (process speed) The phasic alert state
(REA-stab)	The stability of the reaction time	The sustained attention state (repetition 60 times)

The "Symbol-Digit Substitution" (SDS)

This test measurement visual-motor ability (peak performance): The computer screen showed two tables, each containing nine columns and two rows. In the first table, nine geometric forms (shapes) were associated with nine numbers (one digit). The second table showed the same symbols, but in a different order to the first; the subject was required to match the symbols to their corresponding numbers.

TABLE 3.

—	⊥		+	Ǝ	o	U	×	=
1	2	3	4	5	6	7	8	9

⊥	×	—	Ǝ	o		U	=	+

This had to be performed five times with random distribution of symbols in each of the tests.

The software calculated the mean time needed to fill one single cell. The calculations were performed on the best (SDS 1) and second best (SDS 2) series achieved by the subject. Eighteen symbol completions were contained within the two series.

(SDS (1+2)/18) Achieved

Then the software determined the mean time needed to fill a single cell according to the education level and age (only the two best series were taken into account: SDS 1 and SDS 2).

(SDS (1+2)/18 Expected

TABLE 4.

Lb = age of the subject	N = Education level
0 = < than 40 years	1 = Primary school
1 = 40 to 44 years	2 = Secondary school three years
2 = 45 to 49 years	3 = Secondary school six years
3 = 50 to 54 years	4 = Bachelor
4 = >54 years	5 = University master

The calculation of the expected performance was based on this formula:

SDS (1/+2)/18 Expected=2,864 + (0.15) La–0.17N

Then the percentage difference between the expected and achieved values were calculated.

$D\%SDS=(SDS\ (1+2)/18\ Achieved - SDS\ (1+2)/18\ Achieved)/100$

This test evaluated the following functions:

TABLE 5.

	Measure	Evaluate	Includes
Δ%SDS	% variation between expected and achieved mean time needed to fill one cell	Visuo-motor performance	Visual sweeping (and visual field) Visuo-spatial attention

The "Digit Span Backwards" (SDS)

This test was an inverted mnesic span: Several white, five centimeter high, numbers (one digit each) were displayed one by one on a black screen for 0.6 seconds, after which they disappeared. The subject was required to remember them all and enter them in reverse order on a keyboard. The first series was composed of only two numbers; subsequent series increased incrementally by one number until the subject consistently achieved correct scores. The score for the test was the highest level achieved.

The software calculated the mean level (DSB-gem) achieved from:
- Starting level (DSB-start)
- Best level (DSB-max)

The DSB-gem (Expected) was then calculated according to the education level and the subject's age using the following formula:

$DSB\text{-}gem\ (Expected)=4.6 + (2\ x\ 0.3)\ N - 0.5Lb$

TABLE 6.

Lb = age of the subject	N = Education level
0 = < than 40 years	1 = Primary school
1 = 40 to 44 years	2 = Secondary school three years
2 = 45 to 49 years	3 = Secondary school six years
3 = 50 to 54 years	4 = Bachelor
4 = >54 years	5 = University master

Then the percentage variation between DSB-gem (Expected) and DSB-gem (Achieved) was calculated.

$\Delta\%DSB=DSB\text{-}gem\ (Expected) - DSB\text{-}gem\ (Achieved)/100$

The evaluated functions were:

TABLE 7.

	Measure	Evaluate
Δ%DSB	% difference: DSB-gem (Achieved) and DSB-gem (Expected)	Working Memory (WM). Sustained Attention

The "Hand-Eye Coordination" Test (EYE)

A sinusoidal trace was displayed on the screen. The subject was asked to follow this track by means of a cursor moved by the joystick. The subject was only able to control the vertical displacement of the cursor; the sweeping speed (horizontal speed) was set at a constant speed by the computer. After two "test runs," this test was performed seven times.

The software calculated the total surface of the deviations off the proposed track (pixels). The best of the seven series was kept (the least total deviation area performed).

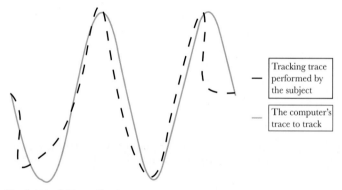

— Tracking trace performed by the subject

— The computer's trace to track

The Evaluated Functions

TABLE 8.

	Measures	Evaluates
EYE-test (pixels)	Total Surface of deviation from the track	Eye-Hand Coordination

The Neuroscreen Scoring

• Scoring of "Simple Reaction Time" (REA) :

Rather than using the simple reaction time, the stability of the simple reaction time (REA-stab) was used to evaluate the test subject (units=milliseconds).

Very Bad	Bad	Insuffient	Normal	Fair	Good	Very Good
> 45	35 to 44.9	30 to 34.9	20 to 29.9	15 to 19.9	10.01 to 14.9	< 10

- Scoring of "Symbol Digit Substitution" (SDS) :
  This test was normalized for the subject's age and education level.
  The measure used was the percentage difference between SDS
  (1+2)/18 Expected and SDS (1+2)/18 Achieved.

Very Bad	Bad	Insuffient	Normal	Fair	Good	Very Good
> +30%	+15 to 30%	+5 to +15%	+5 to -5%	-5 to -15%	-15 to -30%	< to -30%

- Scoring of "Digit Span Backwards" (DSB) :
  This test was classified in the same way as the previous test by
  comparing the "expected" and "achieved" scores; it normalized
  the age and educational level of the subjects.

Very Bad	Bad	Insuffient	Normal	Fair	Good	Very Good
< -30%	-30 to -20%	-19.9 to -10%	-10.1 to +10%	+10.1 to +19.99%	+20 to +30%	> +30%

- Scoring of "Hand-Eye coordination" (EYE) :
  This test was presented as a score: the amount of pixels (area)
  between the target trace and the actual trace performed by
  the subject.

Very Bad	Bad	Normal	Good	Very Good
>5000	5000–3500	3499–2000	2000–1500	< 1500

NEUROPSYCHOMETRIC EVALUATION OUTCOME

The scores obtained by the diver population (n=44) were compared
to the scores in the control group (n=161), and a so-called "pathological"
population who had been exposed to neurotoxic substances (solvents)
(n= 96). Each individual's age and education level was normalized by the

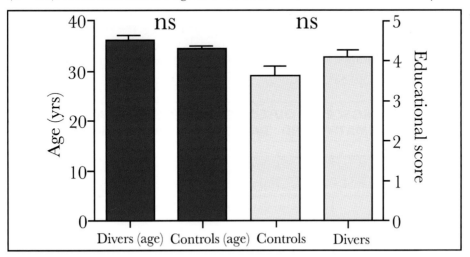

Neuroscreen testing package and thus was not affected by differences
between the population groups.

The Neuroscreen test package had been extensively validated previously
in the field of neurotoxic exposure in industry workers. In fact, an earlier

Figure 1. Matched pairs of divers and controls—age and education comparison.

version of the test (NES) had already been used by another group in the evaluation of divers (Slosman et al., 2004).

As a means of internal validation, divers were "matched" by age (a maximum difference of two years was permitted) and by gender to subjects in the control group. This allowed a parametric comparison between the groups.

Demographics

The group of divers included four female and 38 male divers. One male and one female were excluded due to multiple sclerosis so that a total of 42 were studied. Their mean age was 36.2 years (SD 4.9 years). Mean Body Mass Index (weight/(height)2) was 25.3. Thirty-four (80%) were non-smokers. Mean years diving was 11.7 (SD 6.2). Mean number of dives was 620 (SD 465). Of those, 359 (SD 340) or 57.9% dived shallower than 30 msw; 91 (SD 93) dived deeper than 40 msw. Nineteen of the divers had performed nitrox or trimix dives (45%). For those, a mean of 9% of all dives were performed using mixed gases. Six of the divers (14%) suffered from regular (> 1 per month) migraine attacks. Three (7%) had a history of arterial hypertension; two were on active treatment. As expected, there were no divers who had a history of cardiac or neurological disorders. None had suffered from DCI or even suffered from abnormal fatigue, dizziness, visual or auditory manifestations in relation to diving.

For the general (unmatched) control groups the mean age was 26.5 years (SD 3.5 years); 50% were females. Mean Body Mass Index was 22.4 (SD 3.2). Twenty-three (67%) were regular smokers (mean Pack-Years=5.6).

Neuroscreen Test Results

We compared the scores with non-parametric procedures using Chi square testing (x^2) and Fisher exact test. It was not possible to apply parametric procedures because the raw data did not make provision for the "normalization" process for the various subjects. Accordingly the ordinal outcomes (i.e., very bad, bad, insufficient, fair, normal, good, very good) were compared by calculating the respective proportions of each category and performing non-parametric comparisons.

TABLE 9. NEUROSCREEN OUTCOME FOR RECREATIONAL DIVERS, NORMATIVE AND "PATHOLOGIC" POPULATIONS

Neuroscreen results: Recreational Divers vs. Normative and "Pathological" populations		
Test	**Divers vs. Controls**	**Divers vs. "Pathological's"**
DSB	P<0.001	NS
SDS	P<0.009	NS
REA	NS	P<0.001
EYE	NS	P<0.001

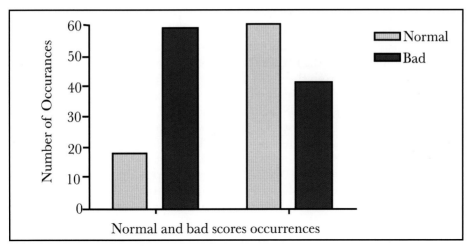

Figure 2. Effect of diving on the Digital Span Backwards.

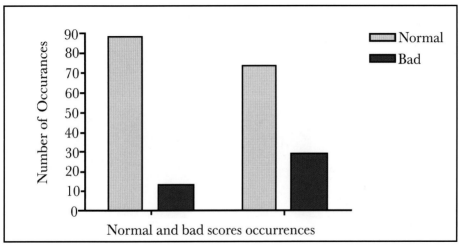

Figure 3. Effect of diving on the SDS Neuroscreen score.

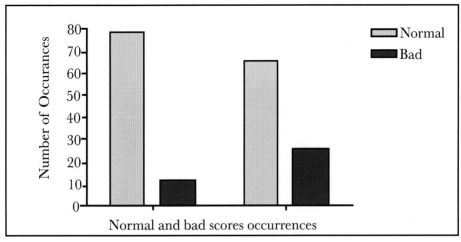

Figure 4. Effect of diving on the simple reaction time stability.

For the Digit-Span Backwards test (DSB), there was a significant difference between the divers and the "normal" population (p=0.001). Surprisingly, the difference between divers and the group "exposed to neurotoxic solvents" was not significant (p=0.442). Both groups performed on average 15–25% worse than expected from the "normal" population results. This test measures the "working memory" and the sustainability of the attention span.

Likewise, for the Symbol-Digit Substitution (SDS), measuring the visual-motor performance (composed of visual sweeping and visual-spatial attention), a significant difference was found between diver and "normal" populations (p<0.0089), but no statistical difference between divers and solvent-exposed controls (p=0.294). Here, both "exposed" groups scored on average 15–30% worse than the "normal" population.

The Simple Reaction Time test (REA) showed a significant difference between the divers and the "normal" population (p=0.626); the divers performed better. The solvent-exposed controls scored significantly worse (p<0.001). The Reaction Time Stability (REA-stab) difference was also in favor of the diving population (p<0.05).

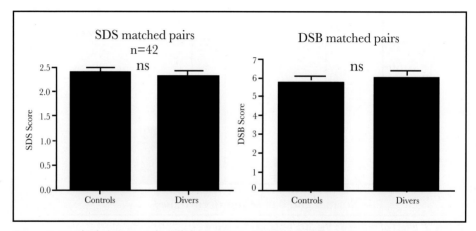

Figure 5. Matched pairs controls and divers SDS and DSB score difference.

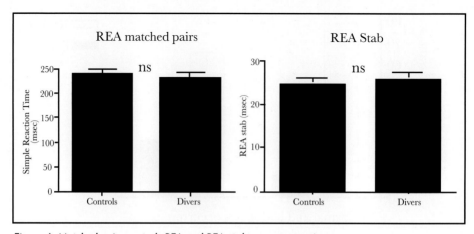

Figure 6. Matched pairs controls REA and REA-stab score comparison.

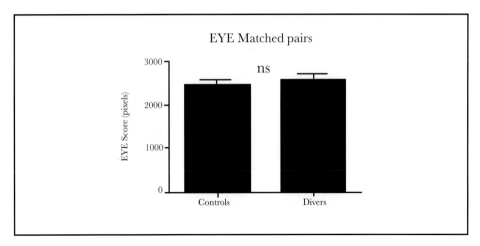

Figure 7. Matched pairs controls EYE score comparison.

The Hand-Eye Coordination Test did not show a significant difference between the divers and the "normal" population (p=0.221) whereas the solvent-exposed controls scored significantly worse (p<0.001).

Comparison with a "Matched" Control Group

Although not required, matched comparisons permitted even better evaluation of the diver's performance.

Correlation between Neuroscreen results and PFO

Patency of the Foramen Ovale was detected in 27 of 42 (64.28%) of the divers, of whom 60% were Grade II PFO (16 divers, 38% of the total). Incomplete fusion of the interatrial septum was detected in 13 divers (30.9%) of whom nine had a Grade II PFO, two a Grade I, and two a Grade 0 PFO. There was no correlation between the presence of PFO and age (r=0.18); number of dives performed (r=0.003); or maneuvers used for middle ear equilibration (r=0.1137). Of the six divers with regular migraine, three had a Grade II PFO, and three were Grade 0.

TABLE 10. NEUROSCREEN OUTCOME FOR PFO VS. NO PFO RECREATIONAL DIVERS

Neuroscreen data comparison between PFO and no PFO recreational divers	
Test	**PFO vs. no-PFO**
DSB	NS
SDS	NS
REA	NS
EYE	NS

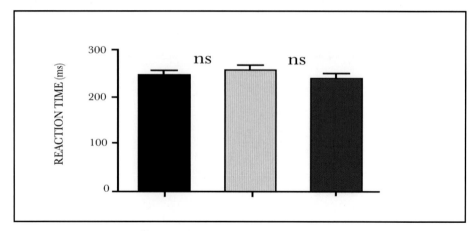

Figure 8. Reaction time and PFO grade comparisons.

The statistical comparison between the c-TEE score for patency of the Foramen Ovale and the Neuroscreen scores for each item did not reach the significance level (X^2) and this was confirmed in the two by two comparisons using the Fisher Exact test. (See table 10)

Sub-group analyzes of the divers with and without PFO showed no significant differences, nor were there any significant differences for divers with Grade II PFO's compared to the rest.

Correlation Between Neuroscreen and Diving Experience

There appeared to be no statistical correlation between the diving experience (number of dives, years of diving) and the neuropsychometric performance. No statistical correlation was found between the mean depth of the dives performed and any of the Neuroscreen items (e.g. REA-stab: r=0.036).

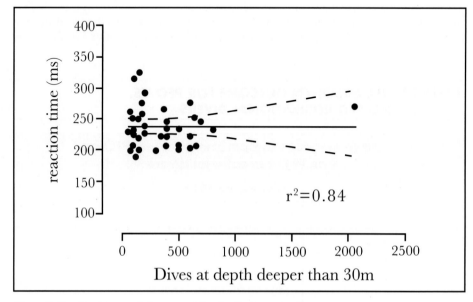

Figure 9. Reaction time and dives over 30m depth regression line.

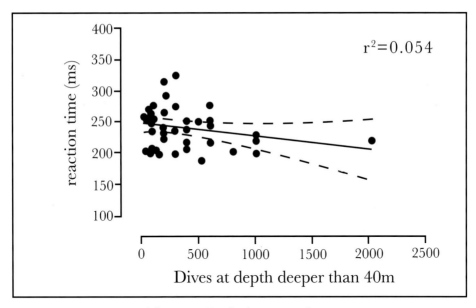

Figure 10. Reaction time and dives over 40m depth regression line.

DISCUSSION

The prevalence of PFO in our diver population was higher than expected from anatomic and cardiologic literature (Hagen et al., 1984; Fisher et al., 1995). There is no clear explanation for this, although it has been suggested from previous studies, personal observations, and one longitudinal follow-up study on PFO (Germonpre et al., 2002), that divers may have a predisposition for "not closing" small PFO's in the course of adult life as other people do (Hagen et al., 1984)—see chapter entitled "Time Related Opening of the Foraman Ovale in Divers." This may lead to a larger than average proportion of divers with large PFO's. Moreover, we have proposed recently that closed or only microscopically patent Foramen Ovale's may be "opened-up" by diving or other strenuous intra-thoracic pressure changing activities (Germonpre et al., 2002). This may be responsible for the almost 65% prevalence in these healthy divers—none of whom have suffered DCI.

Although reported extensively in the literature (Lechat et al., 1989; Bogousslavsky et al., 1996; Anzola et al., 1999; Cujec et al., 1999; Anzola et al., 2000; Wahl et al., 2001; Lamy et al., 2002a; Lamy et al., 2002b; Sztajzel et al., 2002), no specific correlation between PFO and migraine could be detected in our study, although the number of divers with migraine was small (n=6).

The results of our diver population were significantly different from "normal" controls in two of the four tests. However, the divers differed significantly from the "solvent-exposed" control group in the two other tests. Accordingly, we cannot state, "diving is a neuro-toxic agent." For this to be true, all four components would have to be abnormal (Michiels, 1999). However, the impairment of working memory (Thompson-Schill et al., 2002) and visual-spatial skills resembles a milder form of the impairments observed during nitrogen narcosis (Bennett et al., 1981; Edmonds and Boughton, 1985; Michalodimitrakis and Patsalis, 1987; Abraini and Joulia, 1992; Schellart, 1992).

As it is known that nitrogen, as well as other inert gases, exert an influence on a certain membranous neurotransmitter receptors such as dopamine, serotonin and GABA. It is therefore possible to hypothesize that regular diving to "narcotic" depths (more than 30 msw) could diminish, in the long term, the sensitivity of these receptors (Schellart, 1992). This could lead to an ultimate decrement in performance. However, based on our current results, it has not been possible to establish a correlation between the number of dives, number of deep dives, or diving experience in general, vs. the outcome of DSB and SDS testing.

CONCLUSIONS

Using a carefully selected and randomized sample population of recreational divers who have had extensive diving experience without a history or symptoms of DCI; and using a carefully selected, reliable testing technique; we were not able to demonstrate in a conclusive manner any significant neuropsychometric abnormalities in divers as compared to a control group.

There was a distinct and significant deterioration in the neuropsychometric performance in the diver group in the test items measuring working memory and visual-spatial performance. However, it was not possible to define a relationship between patency of the Foramen Ovale, diving experience, and age vs. any of these neuro-psychometric findings.

The similarity of some results in divers and the group exposed to neurotoxic solvents, suggests that there may be some "toxic effects" similar to nitrogen narcosis affecting the divers. This, however, needs to be verified using repeated neuro-psychometric testing to determine if the changes are of a permanent nature.

CHAPTER 12

THE FRACTAL APPROACH AS A TOOL TO UNDERSTAND ASYMPTOMATIC BRAIN HYPERINTENSE MRI SIGNALS

INTRODUCTION

Since the first publication in 1989 that proposed the possible correlation between the presence of a Patent Foramen Ovale (PFO) and the occurrence of decompression illness (DCI) (Moon et al., 1989), there has been much research and speculation on the subject. The Research Department of DAN Europe responded by undertaking a series of studies to address the underlying concerns: "Is there truly an increased risk of DCI for divers who have a PFO?" (Wilmshurst et al., 1986; Wilmshurst et al., 1995; Knauth et al., 1997).

Several years ago two studies appeared that suggested PFO's were associated with cerebral "lesions" in divers (Reul et al., 1995; Knauth et al., 1997). Since then, others have subsequently disputed this direct relationship (Gerriets et al., 2000; Saary and Gray, 2001). The various methodological flaws and difficulties associated with the studies have been considered elsewhere. What remains is the need to determine whether the so-called unidentified bright objects—UBO's—are vascular lesions and consequently possibly related to embolic phenomena.

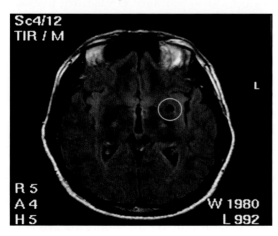

Figure 1. Typical view of a Wirchow-Robin Space with the FLAIR filtering. This is not an abnormal brain spot image.

UBO's are notoriously common, particularly amongst those greater than 40 years of age. Equally plausible, is the over-diagnosis of normal hyperintense areas of the brain visualized by MRI.

To ensure maximum reliability and accuracy, a set of imaging filters was used (T1, T2 and FLAIR sequence) in our study. Particular care was taken in accurately identifying natural lacunar zones known as "Wirchow-Robin spaces" to avoid attributing these to a pathological process (Figure 1). Then, the number and the size of these UBO's found among the divers and non-divers were compared.

In the diver group, the prevalence of cerebral spots was slightly higher than in the non-diver group, but the difference was not significant ($p > 0.05$). This result differs from publications where the diving populations had not been randomized – leaving the possibility of self-selection bias. Given the unanticipated prevalence of 63% PFO's in the diving group, the absence of a significant number of UBO's does not support the proposed correlation between PFO's and UBO's. To further elucidate the possible association, taking into account the non-linear hypothesis of chaos theory, we wanted to analyze the data in a non-linear way.

THE FRACTAL APPROACH

The fractal approach has been developed and used extensively as a mathematical and geometrical assessment tool (Paumgartner et al., 1981; Hastings et al., 1982; Groebe et al., 1990; Hsu and Hsu, 1990; Porter et al., 1991; Meisel, 1992; Keipes et al., 1993; Schindler, 1993; Losa and Nonnenmacher, 1996; Landini, 1997; Maier, 1998; Rigaut et al., 1998; Thill et al., 1998; Chater and Brown, 1999; Peyrin and Guillaume, 1999; Bernard et al., 2001; Mandelbrot et al., 2002). It has enjoyed particular utility in clinical science and pathology (Rossitti, 1995; Sisodiya et al., 1995; Cross, 1997; Caldwell et al., 1998; Handels et al., 1998; Luzi et al., 1999).

In some medical diagnostic fields, fractal analysis appears to offer predictive value–such as in breast cancer (Byng et al., 1996a; Byng et al., 1996b; Velanovich, 1998; Heymans et al., 1999; Zheng and Chan, 2001) and osteoporosis (Feltrin et al., 2001; Dougherty and Henebry, 2002; Lespessailles et al., 2002; Libouban et al., 2002), by analyzing pattern differentiation on the diagnostic images.

The possibility of diagnosis before the appearance of objective findings or clinical symptoms is of paramount importance in modern medicine. For this reason the discovery and use of fractal analysis in neuroimaging is very promising.

Fractal analysis has been used to determine the association between white matter hyperintense "spots" and epileptic seizures in geriatric patients (Takahashi et al., 2001). To our knowledge, however, no investigations have been performed in younger patients to investigate the relation of the fractal dimensions of hyperintense white matter spots in the brain and their spatial distribution. Accordingly, we applied the concept of self-similarity of fractals. We wanted to determine if the fractal dimension of asymptomatic UBO's in divers without DCI or PFO-related headache (Anzola et al., 1999; Wahl et al., 2001; Sztajzel et al., 2002) was compatible with the fractal dimension of the cerebral vasculature. If so, it would increase the probability that UBO's were indeed of vascular origin. Before doing so, we confirmed the reliability of fractal analysis by comparing vascular dimensions to cerebral white spots of known vascular and non-vascular origin respectively. These findings have recently been published (Balestra et al., 2004b).

AN INTRODUCTION TO THE FRACTAL DIMENSION

The term—fractal—comes from word "fraction" (as proposed by B. Mandelbrot) because the general pattern of all structures can be qualified by a fractional approach.

Fractals are characterized by a difference between their topological and fractal dimensions. That is, a fractal line has topological (classic geometrical) dimension of "1," but it could have infinite length and so be space-filling. Its fractal dimension is expressed by an index "μ" (or "D") (the fractal dimension), which for a fractal line takes values $1 \le \mu \le 2$. This abstraction will be shown more clearly by virtue of a well-known example—the "von Koch snowflake" (Mandelbrot, 1983; Trefousse and Vallee, 1991).

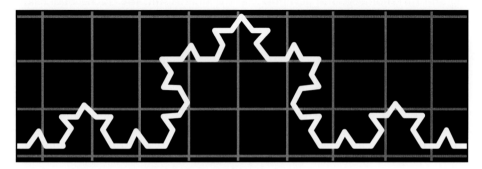

Figure 2. The von Koch snowflake starting image.

This classic fractal possesses a natural ranking of decreasing lengths into distinct scales. Starting from an equilateral triangle with unit side 1, we generate new corners in the middle of each side using a scaling factor $r=1/3$. Subdivide each side into three equal parts, and use the middle section as the basis of an equilateral triangle of side 1/3, pointing outwards. Repeat this process indefinitely. Call the number of divisions=j; number of segments in the entire figure pj and the length of each segment xj. With the initial values $p_0=3$, $x_0=1$, and $L_0=p_0x_0=3$ (total perimeter length of figure), it is easy to show that:

$$p_j = 3 \bullet 4^j, x_j = \frac{1}{3^j}$$

Figure 3.

To avoid confusion, note that here, increasing j corresponds to decreasing x, which is the opposite of other models with scaling. Using (1), the length $L_j = p_j x_j$ (representing the perimeter of the snowflake after j iterations) it becomes infinite as j goes to infinity. The counter-intuitive result of an infinite line enclosed within a finite circle is a consequence of inverse power-law scaling.

On the other hand, the quantity l_n p. l_n x is finite and constant for any j, and is defined as μ, the fractal dimension:

$$\mu = D_H = \frac{\ln 4}{\ln 3} \approx 1.26$$

Figure 4.

Statistical self-similarity (Mandelbrot, 1983), as is found in natural structures, does not give an exact scaling relation. One must not be misled by the high symmetry of the above fractals, as the multiplicity rule is independent of any symmetry.

METHODS

To calculate the fractal dimension of the images we used the Harfa 4.9 (a program applying the modified box counting method after appropriate filtering and thresholding, and accepting, as the final result, the fractal dimension resembling the slope described in the slope analysis option (p<0.001).

Thresholding

The analysis of images needs to perform specific adaptations to be sure to analyze every single image according to the same graphical rules. For instance, the thresholding process is a tool that transforms a color or a grayscale image. The specific parameters of the process can be changed according to the chosen colors (when applicable). In the example an HLS style (Hue-Luminance-Saturation) image is analyzed and the conditions are set to change all pixels to a black color if they meet the following conditions: 1) the HUE values are equal or larger than 81; 2) its brightness is greater or equal to 138; and 3) saturation is greater or equal to 74. All of these conditions have to be fulfilled simultaneously. Pixels that do not fulfill these conditions are changed to white.

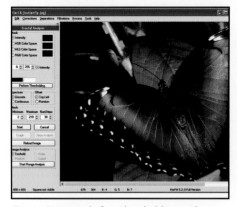

Figure 5. Image before thresholding with specific conditions.

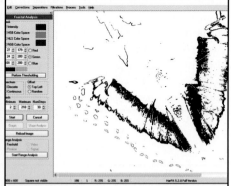

Figure 6. The same image after the specified thresholding.

After proper thresholding, the box counting method can be applied to determine the fractal dimension.

The Box Counting

Traditionally the box counting method is performed by laying meshes of different sizes (r) on the image and particularly on the region of interest (ROI) that is to be measured. The meshes are turned randomly and, each time, the number (N) of boxes needed to cover the object completely is counted. The slope D of the linear portion of the function N *(r)=D (log (1/r)) + log k*, is the fractal dimension and k—the intercept—is the fractal measure. For example if we take a black and white image of a tree:

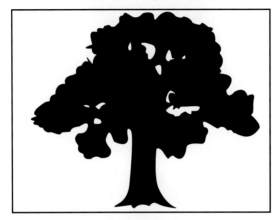

Figure 7. Sample tree image before fractal analysis.

We next overlay it with a mesh of squares sized 10 pixels and then we count the number of squares needed to cover the tree completely, we find that the number of boxes is 520.

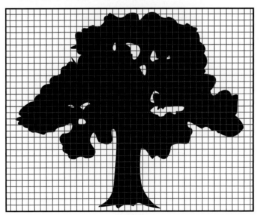

Figure 8. Tree image overlaid with a mesh of 10-pixel squares.

Next, we go on with this process and cover the image with a 17 pixels square box, and find that we need 201 boxes to cover the tree.

Then with another mesh of 28-pixel square boxes (80 boxes needed)

This process should be performed with a sufficient number of steps—for instance, nine steps—then the linear regression can be computed to determine the fractal dimension and the fractal measure. The fractal dimension of the black and white image of the tree is 1.78 with a correlation coefficient R=0.99.

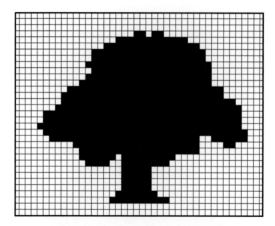

Figure 9. Tree image covered with 520 10-pixel.

Importantly, one must be sure that the fractal dimension chosen is representative of the real trend of the pattern analyzed. As we can see from the graphs, this must be in the linear part of the relation.

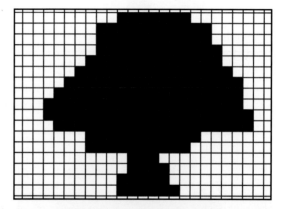

Figure 10. Tree image covered with 17-pixel squares.

The fractality is self-similar and so is scale-independent. Nevertheless, images of fractals are scale-dependent. When the image is enlarged (i.e.,

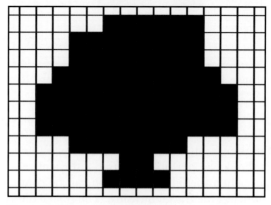

Figure 11. Tree image covered with 28-pixel boxes.

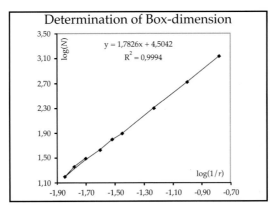

Figure 12. Determination of the fractal dimension.

when the size of the overlying mesh is too small), no fractal but a mosaic composed of white and black elements (pixels) can be seen. If the fractal is reduced too much (i.e., when the squared mesh is too large), the image will disappear in the white background. Distortion can be seen in fractal functions as a disturbance of linearity.

The exact determination of a fractal dimension requires a linear part of the function to be present (Figure 14). To confirm linearity, the correlation coefficients of several data pairs are calculated. The number of data pairs must be large and the span between them is recommended to be at least 20. This means that if we have a set of 100 values we will need to use pairs of values separated in the set by 20 rows; thus, the value number 1 in the set will be paired with the number 21; the number 2 will be paired with the number 22 and so on.

All the pairs will be computed to establish their slope and regression coefficient. The slopes are then reported on a chart (Figure 15) as a function of ln (1/r) of the first value in the segment; the correlation coefficient is color-coded; for instance r=0.999 is coded in red and r > 0.999 is coded in white. The linear part of the function will appear on the graph and distinguish itself

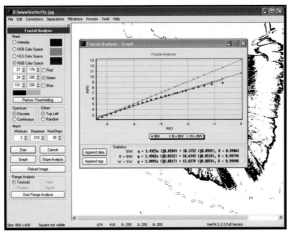

Figure 13. Determination of the fractal dimension for the different edges and colors.

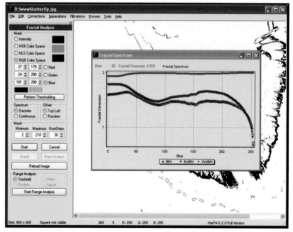

Figure 14. Determination of the fractal dimension for the black and white border.

by a constant part on dependency (the neighbors slopes are nearly the same) and have a high correlation coefficient (0.99 or above).

Population and Data Acquisition

Our population was a group of 42 healthy recreational SCUBA divers under the age of 40. They were selected randomly from a population of 200 volunteer divers based on the following criteria: less than 41 years of age; at least 200 dives; no history of DCI, no evidence of cardiovascular disease, and no other conditions such as multiple sclerosis, migraine or other neurological disease.

MRI images were obtained using a 1.5 Tesla MRI system, with three sequences (axial T2, sagittal T1 and axial FLAIR) in 5mm slices. A "spot" was diagnosed if it appeared at the same time as hyperintense on T2 as well as on FLAIR (Figure 16).

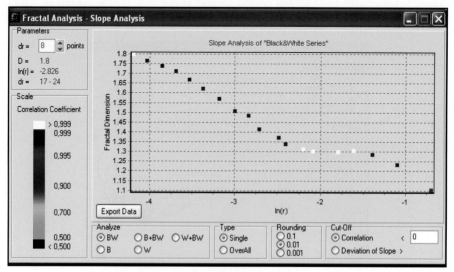

Figure 15. Sample screen of the slope analysis program.

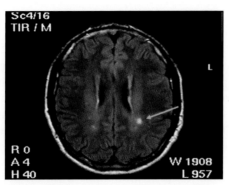

Figure 16. Typical Unidentified Bright Object in a diver's Brain MRI.

MRI images and angiograms from other cerebral pathologies were obtained by electronic means: 18 brain angiographies, 7 MRI images from ischemic (thrombotic) vascular brain lesions, and 9 MRI images of Multiple Sclerosis (Figure 17).

To calculate the fractal dimension of the images we used the Harfa 4.0 program applying the box counting method after appropriated filtering and thresholding and accepting, as the final result, the fractal dimension resembling the slope described in the slope analysis option ($p < 0.001$). Statistical comparison was done with ANOVA testing after Kolmogorov-Smirnov normality compatibility test and Neuman-Keuls discriminating post-test.

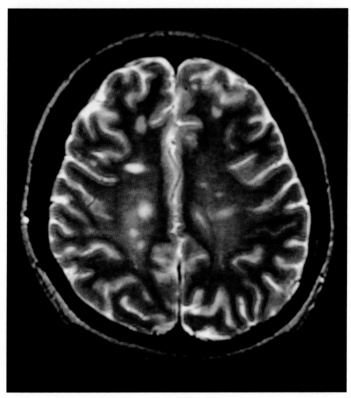

Figure 17. Typical MRI lesions in multiple sclerosis.

RESULTS

In our population of 42 asymptomatic divers, four "lesion-like spots" (UBO's or white matter hyperintense signals) were found. The fractal dimensions of these spots were calculated (D=1,16 +/-0,15) and compared with those of 18 brain angiographies (D=1,67 +/- 0,06). Of those compared, five MRI images were related to thrombotic brain lesions ("vascular images") (D=1,6 +/- 0,05); 9 MRI images of Multiple Sclerosis ("non-vascular images") (D=1,26 +/- 0,13) (Figure 18); 5 MRI images of migraineurs (with aura)–which has been associated with PFO (Anzola et al., 1999; Anzola, 2002; Anzola et al., 2006a; Anzola et al., 2006b); and the 5 asymptomatic scuba divers (i.e., with no DCI history or neurological illnesses—randomized from an population of 200 as described before) with UBO's.

The differences between the fractal dimensions of all the "vascular" images and the diver's "spots" were highly significant (p<0.001). On the other hand, the fractal dimension of "non-vascular" brain lesions was not statistically different from the diver's "spots."

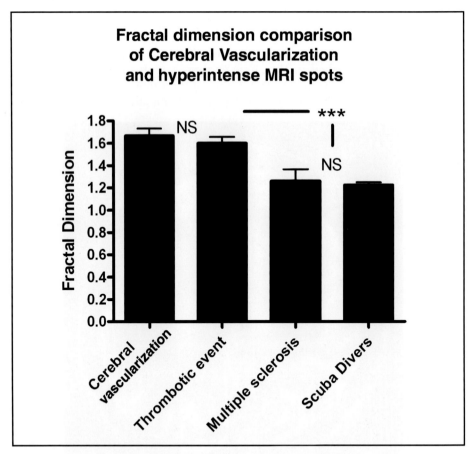

Figure 18 : Fractal Dimension Comparison between different images of cerebral spots (n=22) vs. fractal dimension of normal cerebral angiograms (n=18). Statistical analysis of fractal dimension shows significant differences for multiple sclerosis (n=9) and those found in the scuba divers (n=5) (p<0.001) as opposed to vascular related cerebral spots due to thrombotic stroke (n=5) and migraine with aura (n=5).

As a control, we compared the fractal dimensions of the angiography images (vascular bed spatial distribution) with those of ischemic lesions. No significant statistical difference was found. This indicates that the fractal dimension could accurately discriminate the two different spatial distributions and that it was therefore an appropriate tool for the study.

CONCLUSIONS

We conclude that, using fractal analysis of the MRI "asymptomatic lesions" or UBO's in the brains of divers, these cannot clearly be defined as "vascular" in nature. This observation casts doubt on the ischemic nature of these spots. As a corollary observation, the link between the patency of the Foramen Ovale of the heart and these diver's "spots" is not as clear as has been postulated (Knauth et al., 1997; Schwerzmann and Seiler, 2001). However, migraine with aura is associated with PFO, and PFO closure appears to mitigate these events (Anzola et al., 1999; Anzola, 2002; Anzola et al., 2006a; Anzola et al., 2006b). While there are recent non-shunting-related theories for migraine with aura (Yetkin et al., 2006), our findings support the former hypotheses. Nevertheless, cerebral spots in asymptomatic divers with PFO were not associated with a vascular distribution and, accordingly, their relation to diving should be questioned based on our current understanding of decompression pathophysiology of the brain.

NOTES

CHAPTER 13

GENERAL CONCLUSIONS

ACCORDING TO OUR RESULTS THE FOLLOWING CONCLUSIONS CAN BE DRAWN:

Prevalence of PFO in divers

The prevalence of patency of the Foramen Ovale is greater in divers who have experienced an episode of cerebral decompression illness. This prevalence is clear when we look at the association between cerebral DCI symptoms and the presence of Grade II PFO's. The statistical power is assured using a matched pair, controlled, retrospective study.

PFO prospective screening

A prospective study design is required to study the relative risk of developing DCI as a diver with a PFO. This requires a large number volunteers and a low-risk, minimally invasive, reliable screening procedure. The Carotid Doppler screening procedure has been compared to the Gold Standard of PFO detection (TEE) in a randomized population. It carries 100% sensitivity. Due to the inability to differentiate pulmonary shunts, CD has a slightly lower specificity. An international prospective multicenter study is ongoing and the first results are anticipated in 2008.

Intrathoracic pressure variations

The mechanisms influencing the passage of blood (and venous gas bubbles) through a PFO have been studied by measuring the changes in intrathoracic pressure resulting from a number of procedures used to elicit shunting (opening a PFO). Our results suggest that the primary determinant of interatrial pressure reversal is the duration of the increase in intrathoracic pressure and not the absolute pressure per se. The "diver's" Valsalva maneuver—as used during normal ear equalization—produces neither the duration nor the significant increases in intrathoracic pressure required for interatrial pressures reversal.

Methodological aspects

A thorough review of the available literature shows that most published research reports do not take into account the duration of the provocative respiratory maneuvers used during the c-TEE screening procedure. As a result, false negatives may lead to an underestimation of PFO patency. It is recommended to sustain the increase in intrathoracic pressure for at least six to ten seconds in order to provoke significant pressure reversal with shunting upon release. As the consequences of this methodological flaw would be an underestimation of PFO, earlier studies may need to be re-evaluated or even repeated.

Time-related opening

Having established a standardized methodology and semi quantification of PFO patency, we retested several volunteers a few years after the first examination to determine variations in patency. We made the unexpected finding of an increase in patency over time; some de nuovo patencies; and one spontaneous closure of a previous PFO. It appears that PFO's are not static so that a single examination can neither predict long-term patency nor exclude the possibility of spontaneous closure. The explanation for these phenomena is still being researched.

MRI UBO's and PFO's in divers

Several studies on the long term neurological effects of diving have reported hyperintense spots in MRI brain images of divers and have suggested that these represent long-term damage as a result of diving. However, a closer look at most of the experimental protocols has revealed several methodological flaws such as self-selection bias. We performed a randomized, controlled study that was unable to attribute UBO's to diving or the presence of PFO when the results were compared to matched non-diving controls. The only significant finding was that the mean size of UBO's appeared to be greater in the diving group.

Psychometric evaluation of divers

Following the finding that divers had larger UBO's than non-divers, we wanted to determine if this had any clinical implications. We chose a computer-administered, extensively validated, psychometric testing battery: the Neuroscreen test. We compared the results to a control group and to a group who had suffered occupational exposure to neurotoxic agents. The Neuroscreen test consists of four components. We were able to document a statistical difference between divers and controls on two of the items. The same two items were not statistically different from the exposed group. However, these results did not support the hypothesis that sport diving was associated with long-term neurological sequelae. Abnormality in all four items would be required for such a conclusion. Nevertheless, this is an important area for further research.

The Fractal approach as a tool to understand diver's MRI UBO's

For UBO's to be considered the consequences of paradoxical embolization, they would need to be associated with cerebral vasculature. In lieu of histological examination, it is possible to analyze the spatial distribution of such spots and compare it to the spatial distribution of the cerebral vascular bed using fractal analysis. After validating this approach by comparing the mean values of the fractal dimension of images coming from clearly vascular (angiography and thrombotic cerebral vascular episodes) to clearly non-vascular cerebral spots images (multiple sclerosis MRI), and then comparing all of them to the images obtained from divers, it was possible to conclude that UBO's in divers were not associated with vascular lesions. Therefore, as a general conclusion, it cannot be said that PFO is a sole risk factor for DCI. It has to be kept in mind that DCI is multifactorial and may depend more on the volume of circulating bubbles than a PFO. Our conclusions do not suggest that divers with a PFO should not dive, but rather that all divers should follow a "no bubbles no problems" approach. This may be achieved by taking additional precautions during the ascent—such as possibly including additional deep stops on dives in excess of 25 m (Marroni et al., 2004b). This is considered in greater detail in the next chapter.

NOTES

CHAPTER 14

SAFER DECOMPRESSION AND LOW BUBBLE PRODUCTION PROCEDURES

The origins of modern understanding of decompression are founded on the principles set by Haldane in 1908 (Boycott et al., 1908). These mathematical approximations of physiological phenomena–also called classic or "Haldanian" models—form the basis of most military, commercial and recreational diving tables in use today. All share the same fundamental principles:

- That inert gas exchange may be represented by a series of exponential compartments; and that,
- Safe return to the surface is dependent on avoiding critical saturation in any of these compartments.

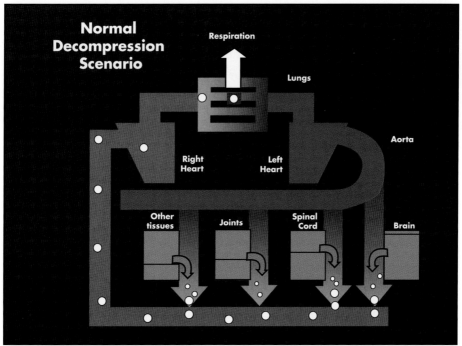

Figure 1. The consequences of "normal" decompression—venous gas emboli without tissue bubbles.

Although decompression procedures and tables have been modified many times since scuba diving was initiated as a sport in 1943, and in spite of the current prevalence of dive computers assisting with decompression, the incidence of decompression sickness (DCI) has changed very little (Landsberg, 1976; Dembert, 1977; Steinbruck and Paeslack, 1980; Calder, 1985; Murrison et al., 1991; Gallagher, 1997). This may be because these modifications have not addressed all the critical variables for safe decompression.

Most decompression models have relied on Haldane's hypothesis of "tissue" exponentials—typically 5, 10, 20, 40, 80 and 120 minute halftimes (Hempelman, 1993). Traditionally, the first three were considered fast tissue compartments and the last three "slow." For each of these compartments, a critical saturation ratio was defined, that is, the limit was defined by which inert gas in each compartment could exceed ambient pressure without producing bubbles. In the original Haldane model, this ratio was 2:1 for all tissues. However, practical experience eventually softened ratios on fast tissues while lowering those in slow tissues. As a result, fast tissues no longer controlled the ascent on many dive profiles. However, given the fact that 65% of DCI cases in recreational divers are neurological—i.e., related to fast tissues—the wisdom of these modifications is again being questioned.

Neurological DCI is often related to the spinal cord. Nearly half of these events do not seem to be due to a violation of decompression tables. With spinal cord tissue having an estimated half time of only 12.5 minutes (Edmonds et al., 1992), a typical 25-meter (100 feet) dive of 25 minutes would saturate this tissue compartment by at least 75%. The logical conclusion must be that this tissue somehow controls the ascent from these dives, even though modern algorithms and computers de-emphasize its importance. Consequently, more stops may be required to desaturate fast tissues in an effort to avoid neurological DCI.

Interestingly, the original Haldane table for a 25 meters/25 minute dive required decompression stops at nine, six and three meters with a total decompression time of 19 minutes (Hempleman et al., 1984; Hempelman, 1993). Yet today, with an ascent of 30 feet per minute and a "safety stop" at 15 feet for three minutes, the diver is on the surface in only some six minutes; this may be far too short for adequate desaturation of these tissue compartments. Not surprisingly, deep stops have recently been proposed for deeper recreational diving. The origin of deep stops lies buried in a bit of decompression history that has somehow been lost over the past century.

The original research by Haldane with goats maintained that for a dive to an absolute pressure of P_1, the absolute pressure reduction during decompression—to P_2—should not be more than half the pressure of P_1. This 2:1 ratio of Haldane is widely quoted even though it was *not actually used* in his later decompression tables. In contrast, Leonard Hill believed in slow linear ascent (Valentine, 2000). However, experiments with goats ultimately confirmed that Haldane's method of decompression was superior. Hill's method of slow linear ascent was not effective and resulted in DCI. Ironically, today, for no decompression-stop diving, a linear ascent rate of between 9 and 18 meters per minute is recommended—depending on the tables. Even though the lower rates are now almost universally recommended, the ascent remains linear.

When it was found that even this strategy did not eliminate DCI, a single brief safety stop at five meters (15 feet) was recommended, from where the diver would then surface—usually far too rapidly. Modifications to the Haldane model by the US Navy had the effect of eliminating the need for more decompression stops during ascent. Consequently, the so-called 'deep stop' was lost.

Interestingly, many native diving communities that have developed their own empirical diving techniques, have spontaneously introduced "deep stops" to avoid a high incidence of DCI (Wong, 2003).

IDENTIFYING THE RISK OF DECOMPRESSION ILLNESSES

Although it is intuitive to determine the relative safety of decompression tables by measuring the incidence of decompression sickness (Balldin, 1980; Arness, 1997; Ball et al., 1999; Carturan et al., 1999; Carturan et al., 2002) the matter is not that simple. The relatively low incidence of decompression illnesses, the ambiguity of symptoms, and the absence of any objective diagnostic tools, make this a challenging task.

The introduction of diving injury databases in the 70–80's, and also more recent epidemiological research initiatives by Divers Alert Network, has provided at least some information for statistical analysis (Imbert and Montbaron, 1990; Imbert, 1993). DCI symptoms include a wide span of problems ranging from mild skin rash or articular pain to severe neurological symptoms and even death. The various classification systems for DCI, and their respective limitations, have been discussed in detail in the chapter entitled "An Introduction to Clinical Aspects of Decompression Illness." What remains is to determine whether certain dive profiles predisposes to a higher incidence or a greater severity of DCI.

In the 1974 edition of the Comex Medical Book, Dr. X Fructus differentiated between vestibular hits and other neurological symptoms. Following the outcome of his early work on bounce diving using his decompression tables, called the Cx70 tables, he came to suspect that different dive profiles predisposed to different neurological manifestations. Unpublished safety records from the North Sea Comex Database, showed that there was an uneven distribution of risk over the wide range of pressure-time exposures (Imbert and Montbaron, 1990). Long bottom times (90–120 minutes) tended to induce joint and skin problems. Intermediate bottom times (30–60 minutes), on the other hand, preferentially produced neurological symptoms–either central or spinal. Surprisingly, very short bottom times (10–30 minutes) exclusively produced vestibular symptoms.

Typical of their time, the Cx70 tables were characterized by a long haul from the bottom to the first stop–performed at a rapid initial ascent rate. This was particularly significant for short bottom times. For instance, a particular concern was the 66 meter/20 minute table with a first stop at 12 meters, leading to an initial ascent

---

† The lessons learned from the Cx70 tables are of particular importance to technical divers. The divers usually have 15 to 20 minute bottom times making a vestibular hit more likely. This is a serious accident, not only because of the hazards associated with the ensuing disorientation, nausea, and vomiting underwater, but also because this condition has proven to be particularly refractory to treatment. Because of this threat of symptoms occurring in the water, technical divers must use very conservative tables.

of 54 meters over 3 minutes at 18 meters per minute. Safety analysis of these early deep bounce tables clearly showed that this profile was hazardous. In later revisions, the initial ascent phase was slowed down significantly [†].

STRATEGIES FOR SUCCESSFUL DECOMPRESSIONS

Through time and experience, divers have continued to modify decompression schedules empirically for the purposes of achieving greater safety. Shorter bottom times, longer stops, and slower ascent rates have been the primary three strategies.

Several years ago, recreational divers adopted the empirical "safety stop," at three to five meters for three to five minutes, as an additional arbitrary safety measure. More recently, there has been an increasing trend to introduce a so-called deep stop during the ascent from deeper dives. A lovely anecdote to this effect is the tale by a pair of 50-something coral hunters who decided to stop halfway during their ascent from deep dives to sing a hymn. They added, with a smile, that they adapted the number of verses depending on how comfortable they felt during the decompression. While hardly scientific, the principle behind the decision was not entirely ill conceived.

Deep stops are not a new phenomenon. They already appeared in the early editions of the Royal Navy diving manual. This manual included a set of deep air tables to 90 meters, which boasted a decompression stop at half the depth. Deep stops were also recommended by Richard Pyle in articles published in the "Deep Tech" diving magazines (Pyle, 1999). Being an ichthyologist by occupation, Pyle discovered that he was required to perform a deep stop after collecting fish at greater depths for the Hawaii Aquarium. He found that if he stopped halfway during the ascent and punctured the swim bladder with a needle, the fish would arrive at the surface in better condition. As it turned out—so did he! Both he and his entire dive team felt far less tired after including the deep stops for the sake of the fish.

MEDITERRANEAN CORAL DIVING

Red coral jewels are a traditional commodity around the Mediterranean. Coral has been collected for centuries by dragging an assembly of beams and nets, called "the cross," along the underwater walls. This has largely contributed to the destruction of shallow coral outcrops. As a result, collection dives are now deeper and collecting methods more precise.

Since the introduction of SCUBA diving, there has been a small population of coral divers in France, mainly along the Côte d'Azur and in Corsica, who pursue these creatures for a living. Diving for coral is tough; during the season divers perform two 20-minute dives per day to depths of 80–90 meters on air. Recently, because coral is getting even scarcer, divers have had to start using trimix (oxygen, nitrogen and helium mixtures) enabling them to work around 100–130 meters.

Coral divers use a variety of empirical decompression procedures based on experience; they are loath to share their secrets, however. Typically they use one set of decompression stops for a range of exposures, all learned by heart. They usually carry their bottom breathing gas mixture in two or three cylinder configurations, and then rely on gas supply from the surface to support them during their final ascent. They also use oxygen aggressively during decompression, usually starting at 12 or even 15 meters in water. Some of them use a decompression chamber on board the dive vessel and perform surface decompression. Coral dive tables are dramatically shorter than the equivalent commercial or recreational schedules. Accordingly, they must be doing something differently to escape without injury. The following is common practice: after completing their bottom time, coral divers rapidly ascend by 10–15 meters to reduce the narcosis. Then they slow down their ascent to between six and nine meters per minute until they reach 40 meters. Here they wait for the boat to spot their surface bubbles. When the boat is positioned above them, they send a lift bag to the surface with the coral basket

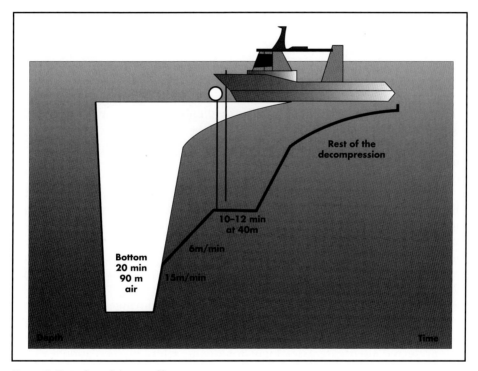

Figure 2. Typical coral diver profile.

attached to one end. The crew then send them the decompression gas line (called an umbilical) using the same line. When the basket is secured, the divers proceed with the rest of their decompression. This way, the dive profile is lengthened by some 8–10 minutes, spent at mid depth, and apparently essential for their safe decompression.

COMEX DEEP DECOMPRESSION STUDIES

In 1977, Comex commercial diving company was planning large-scale deep diving operations and wanted to select a pool of divers based on their resistance to High Pressure Nervous Syndrome (HPNS). As the speed of compression is an important risk factor for HPNS, the divers were pressurized to 180 meters in 15 minutes. Upon reaching the bottom, they were subjected to a two-hour psychomotor test battery after which they were decompressed.

Bernard Gardette, who was charged with calculating the decompression procedures (Gardette, 1979, 1989), experienced great difficulties in developing a mathematical model for such severe exposure. He finally gave up the idea of any mathematical support and simply started drawing the decompression profiles on paper. After some trials, he discovered that by plotting the ascent rate on a logarithm scale vs. depth on a linear scale, decompressions roughly resembled a straight line. Using his findings to design a set of decompression tables, he produced decompressions with varying rates of ascent and very deep stops. After some adjustments, he eventually completed a schedule for the 180 meter/120 minute dive; it required 48 hours of decompression and appeared extremely safe. A total of 49 divers went through the selection tests without any symptoms (Gardette, 1979). The characteristic of the semi-log plot is that it expanded the deeper portion of the decompression and made it possible to define rates of ascent in an area where traditional models failed to control the ascent rate on pressure ratios. For example, a Haldane model would have permitted nearly instantaneous ascent from 180–75 meters on the 2:1 principle. Although the method was deliberately empirical, it gave varying initial ascent rates that progressively turned into short deep stops.

The French Navy, who attempted to design similar deep bounce tables in the 150–180 meter range only succeeded in bringing the divers safely back to surface by using a near-saturation decompression profile.

It is evident from all this that there are two primary conflicting objectives during ascent: 1) increasing pressure gradients so as to eliminate inert gas more quickly, yet 2) avoiding excessive bubble formation in the process. Appropriate combinations of ascent rates and stops should afford the optimal benefit of both–the so-called *economy of decompression*. This has become a major stimulus for research by DAN Europe and others in the context of recreational diving.

The practical difficulty of monitoring bubbles during ascent has made way to immediate, post-dive, precordial Doppler bubble assessment. Post-decompression bubble detection, rather than DCI incidence, has now become the preferred surrogate assessment for diving safety in recreational divers who dive within traditional boundaries of safe decompression.

In an effort to better delineate the respective safety factors, we have designed an ongoing series of studies—both in open water and in decompression chambers—to address the following questions, hypotheses, and concerns:

- Is there a benefit to slowing ascent rate prior to the first stop?
- Should ascent rates be faster or slower than is currently recommended?
- Should deeper decompression stops be introduced? If so, on which dives?
- Does an empirical stop at half-the-depth offer a benefit during ascent?
- How should these various factors be combined?

CHAPTER 15

THE ARTERIAL BUBBLE ASSUMPTION

Although decompression bubbles are primarily venous, (i.e., venous gas emboli), the idea of arterial bubbles was already contained in the seminal paper by Haldane in 1908:

"If small bubbles are carried through the lung capillaries and pass, for instance, to a slowly desaturating part of the spinal cord, they will there increase in size and may produce serious blockage of circulation or direct mechanical damage."

More recently, in 1971, Hills was able to show—using an animal model — that DCI symptoms could change from minor to severe by changing from continuous to surface decompression (Hills, 1971). This elegant experiment demonstrated the existence of a different mechanism for the onset of so-called type III DCI that was later accounted for by arterial bubbles.

Our findings do not suggest that arterial bubbles are common during decompression. Moreover, we have found no associated evidence for the asymptomatic cerebral MRI findings reported in divers with PFO's where a

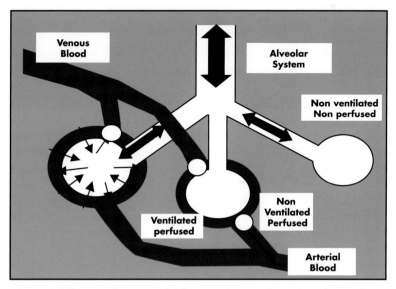

Figure 1. Schematic illustration of pulmonary shunts and paradoxical arterial gas embolism.

history of DCI is absent. However, there does indeed appear to be an association between PFO and cerebral DCI, and here paradoxical embolism appears more likely (Germonpré et al., 1996; Germonpre et al., 1998a). The role of the pulmonary "bubble trap," and whether or not its failure may contribute significantly to paradoxical embolism, remains a source of uncertainty (Cooke et al., 1976; Butler & Hills, 1979; Brubakk et al., 1986; Dujic et al., 1992; Heritier et al., 1993; Butler, 1996). Our results suggest that at least 10% of the population may have pulmonary shunts that could permit venous gas emboli to become arterial—as detected by carotid Doppler (Blatteau, 1999; Germonpré et al., 1999; Balestra et al., 2000a). The possibility of alveola

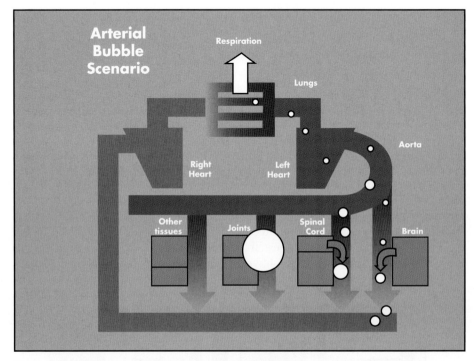

Figure 2. The destination of paradoxical arterial gas embolism.

micro-trauma during a normal ascent with AGE should be entertained when shunting has been excluded.

To bypass pulmonary capillaries, bubbles are required to have the size of a red blood cell (+/- 7μm). This suggests that a diagnostic procedure designed to identify such passage would require the injection of gas bubbles of roughly the same size. Recently an interesting study using "Levovist," an injected vascular ultrasound contrast, has confirmed that these three to eight micron bubbles could circulate freely throughout the body in all tested subjects (Besnard, 2002). It could therefore similarly be hypothesized that very tiny inert gas bubbles could pass to the arterial side, particularly during the initial phases of decompression, when surrounding tissues are not significantly supersaturated and the bubbles would remain small. By the time of such bubbles become detectable by Doppler, they are between 20 and 30 microns in diameter and would no longer be able to traverse normal pulmonary capillaries. Therefore, it is important to realize that post-diving precordial Doppler is not likely to be a useful screening tool for arterial embolization.

Importantly, there is increasing evidence supporting the hypothesis that microparticles and other vasoactive mediators may be responsible for vascular reactions rather than specific bubble occlusive events. Consequently, this de-emphasizes the need for arterial bubbles to explain certain vascular and neurological decompression pathologies. Venous gas emboli—while possibly within the threshold of critical volume and in the absence of shunting—may therefore nevertheless precipitate the release of vasoactive substances resulting in systemic pathological processes that would otherwise be attributed to the arterialization of bubbles (Klinkner et al., 2006; Morel et al., 2006a; Morel et al., 2006b; Piccin et al., 2006; Simak et al., 2006).

In closing, rather than being preoccupied with bubble shunting, we should perhaps afford greater importance to the reduction of all bubbles thereby reducing their global effects on vascular function. The concept of a better *economy of decompression* i.e., expedient decompression without any significant bubble production—is therefore likely to remain a primary objective in the years to come.

NOTES

CHAPTER 16

GENERAL CONCLUSIONS, FINAL REMARKS

The current incidence of DCI is relatively stable despite various empirical modifications to bottom time, ascent rates and the introduction of diving computers. The incidence remains around 0.026% for the DCI occurrences and around 0.12% (2006 DAN data) for minor events; a very low incidence when compared to other diving procedures (Marroni et al., 1983).

The reason for this relative stability may be pervading deficiencies in our decompression algorithms to model with sufficient accuracy the specific physiological events that occur during decompression, or it may be that some individuals have unique biological sensitivity to bubbles and their pathophysiological effects. It is our hope that ongoing field studies may enable us to close the gaps in our understanding. The DAN Europe Dive Safety Laboratory and DAN America Project Dive Safety programs have been very helpful in doing just that. The current DAN Europe Dive Safety Laboratory data consist of more than 38,000 recreational dive profiles of which more than 2,500 also have Doppler data (see Figure 58). So far, ten DCI incidents have been recorded—an inci-

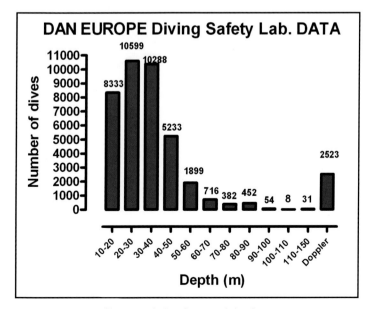

Figure 1. Dive profiles recorded in the actual database.

dence of 0.026%. Interestingly, none of the ten decompression injuries were "deserved and expected" according to the decompression algorithm/dive computers used by the divers, but the analysis of the dive profiles showed tissue saturation levels compatible with high grade bubble formation according to our studies (see below).

The analysis of the previous data in Figure 1 has shown:

- The occurrence of bubbles in recreational diving is more common than previously believed (+/- 30% in the first dive and 67% in repetitive dives) (Marroni et al., 1996; Marroni et al., 2000).
- Avoidance of significant quantities of circulating venous gas appears to be a critical factor in further improvements in decompression safety. Irrespective of whether venous gas bubbles become arterialized (i.e., due to a PFO or pulmonary shunt) or precipitate the release of vasoactive mediators / microparticles, the avoidance of venous gas emboli remains the primary method of prevention.
- The cooling of the skin seems related to bubble production after diving (Marroni et al., 2001a).
- Precordial Doppler scores tend to peak (i.e., the number of venous gas emboli are highest) 25 to 75 minutes after surfacing for repetitive and single dives respectively (Figure 2).
- Controlling fast tissue saturation seems to be essential to successful decompression procedures in recreational diving (Marroni et al., 2001c).
- The First Delta P seems to be a primary factor in the production of bubbles: Calculated venous N_2 pressure should not exceed 1100 mbars and the M value of the fast tissues should not exceed 80% of the predicted maximum (Marroni et al., 2002b).

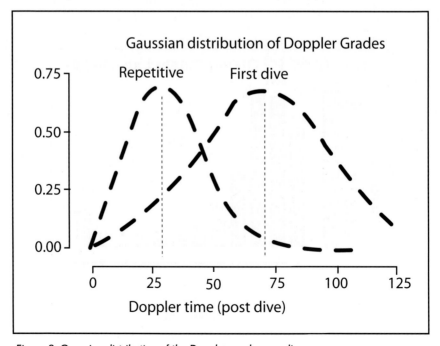

Figure 2. Gaussian distribution of the Doppler grade recordings.

- The rate of ascent is important, but the depth and duration of stops appear to make a great impact on the ultimate precordial Doppler scores (Marroni et al., 2001b).
- By reducing the M-value of the fast compartments and by introducing deep stops, circulating venous gas can virtually be eliminated after diving (Marroni et al. 2001c).
- Deep stops, when employed empirically in a "normal" (no decompression) recreational dive profile (Pyle, 1999), appear to drastically reduce bubble production after single or repetitive diving (Marroni et al., 2002a).

The general conclusions of our study are that less emphasis should be placed on the patency of cardiac foramen ovale as an independent risk factor for DCI, and that more effort and research should be spent on reducing venous gas bubble production through:

- the optimal combination of ascent rates and stops i.e., better economy of decompression with the objective — no bubbles, no troubles!
- by reducing the formation and migration of bubbles within the body by reducing endothelial morphological causes of bubble formation as well as situations where bubble shunting is likely to occur; and finally
- by reducing the body's response to the direct and indirect effects of bubbles on endothelial function due to the release of vasoactive particles.

These avenues of research are likely to lead to new recommendations on diving methods in the future. However, for the moment, in spite of all the theoretical concerns for the health and safety of divers, scuba diving remains a safe and enjoyable sport and nothing in our work suggests otherwise.

NOTES

SECTION 3
REFERENCES

REFERENCES

Aarli JA, Vaernes R, Brubakk AO, Nyland H, Skeidsvoll H, Tonjum S. (1985). Central nervous dysfunction associated with deep-sea diving. *Acta Neurol Scand* 71, 2-10.

Abraini JH, Joulia F. (1992). Psycho-sensorimotor performance in divers exposed to six and seven atmospheres absolute of compressed air. *Eur J Appl Physiol Occup Physiol* 65, 84-87.

Anzola GP. (2002). Clinical impact of patent foramen ovale diagnosis with transcranial Doppler. *Eur J Ultrasound* 16, 11-20.

Anzola GP, Del Sette M, Rozzini L, Zavarise P, Morandi E, Gandolfo C, Angeli S, Finocchi C. (2000). The migraine-PFO connection is independent of sex. *Cerebrovasc Dis* 10, 163.

Anzola GP, Frisoni GB, Morandi E, Casilli F, Onorato E. (2006a). Shunt-associated migraine responds favorably to atrial septal repair: a case-control study. *Stroke* 37, 430-434.

Anzola GP, Magoni M, Guindani M, Rozzini L, Dalla Volta G. (1999). Potential source of cerebral embolism in migraine with aura: a transcranial Doppler study. *Neurology* 52, 1622-1625.

Anzola GP, Morandi E, Casilli F, Onorato E. (2006b). Different degrees of right-to-left shunting predict migraine and stroke: data from 420 patients. *Neurology* 66, 765-767.

Arness MK. (1997). Scuba decompression illness and diving fatalities in an overseas military community. *Aviat Space Environ Med* 68, 325-333.

Augusseau MP, Pacouret G, Charbonnier B, Sirinelli A, Dreyfus X, Aupart M. (1997). [Paradoxical embolism and thrombosis trapped in the foramen ovale. Role of trans-esophageal echocardiography]. *Arch Mal Coeur Vaiss* 90, 1533-1538.

Balestra C. (2000). Patent Foramen Ovale as a risk factor for Extravehicular Spatial Activities, pp. 1-89. NASA, Houston (Tx-USA).

Balestra C, Germonpré P, Kitoko L, Unger P, Snoeck T, Salem W. (2000a). Carotid Artery Doppler as a Screening Method for Patency of the Foramen Ovale. *Sport Geneeskunde & Sport Wetenschappen* 83, 21-23.

Balestra C, Germonpré P, Kitoko L, Unger P, Snoeck T, Salem W. (2000b). Carotid Artery Doppler as a Screening method for patency of the Foramen Ovale. In *Belgisch Verniging voor Sportgeneeskunde en Sportwetenschappen,* ed. Meuusen R, pp. 15. Brussel (VUB).

Balestra C, Germonpre P, Marroni A. (1998). Intrathoracic pressure changes after Valsalva strain and other maneuvers: implications for divers with patent foramen ovale. *Undersea Hyperb Med* 25, 171-174.

Balestra C, Germonpre P, Snoeck T, Ezquer M, Leduc A, Leduc O, Willeput F, Marroni A, Cali Corleo R, Vann R. (2004a). Normobaric oxygen can enhance protein captation by the lymphatic system in healthy humans. *Undersea Hyperb Med* 31, 59-62.

Balestra C, Germonpré P, Snoeck T, Marroni A, Cali Corleo R, Farkas B. (2002). PFO Detection in Divers - Methodological aspects. *European Journal of Underwater and Hyperbaric Medicine* 3, 74.

Balestra C, Germonpré P, Vanderschueren F, Heyters C, Hotton R, Oz S. (1996). Intrathoracic pressure falls after Valsalva manoeuvre and isometric exercise are identical: implications for divers with patent foramen Ovale. In *International Joint Meeting on Hyperbaric Medicine*, ed. Wattel F, Oriani G, Marroni A, pp. 89-90. Galeazzi Hyperbaric Institute, Milano, (Italy).

Balestra C, Marroni A, Farkas B, Peetrons P, Vanderschueren F, Duboc E, Snoeck T, Germonpre P. (2004b). The Fractal Approach as a Tool to Understand Asymptomatic Brain Hyperintense MRI Signals. *Fractals* 12, 67-72.

Ball R, Lehner CE, Parker EC. (1999). Predicting risk of decompression sickness in humans from outcomes in sheep. *J Appl Physiol* 86, 1920-1929.

Balldin UI. (1980). Venous gas bubbles while flying with cabin altitudes of airliners or general aviation aircraft 3 hours after diving. *Aviat Space Environ Med* 51, 649-652.

Bartzokis G, Beckson M, Hance DB, Lu PH, Foster JA, Mintz J, Ling W, Bridge P. (1999a). Magnetic resonance imaging evidence of "silent" cerebrovascular toxicity in cocaine dependence. *Biol Psychiatry* 45, 1203-1211.

Bartzokis G, Goldstein IB, Hance DB, Beckson M, Shapiro D, Lu PH, Edwards N, Mintz J, Bridge P. (1999b). The incidence of T2-weighted MR imaging signal abnormalities in the brain of cocaine-dependent patients is age-related and region-specific. *AJNR Am J Neuroradiol* 20, 1628-1635.

Belkin RN, Pollack BD, Ruggiero ML, Alas LL, Tatini U. (1994). Comparison of transesophageal and transthoracic echocardiography with contrast and color flow Doppler in the detection of patent foramen ovale. *Am Heart J* 128, 520-525.

Benestad HB, Hersleth IB, Hardersen H, Molvaer OI. (1990). Functional capacity of neutrophil granulocytes in deep-sea divers. *Scand J Clin Lab Invest* 50, 9-18.

Bennett PB, Coggin R, Roby J. (1981). Control of HPNS in humans during rapid compression with trimix to 650 m (2131 ft). *Undersea Biomed Res* 8, 85-100.

Bennett PB, Elliott DH. (1993). *The Physiology and medicine of diving*. Saunders, London; Philadelphia.

Bergh K, Hjelde A, Iversen OJ, Brubakk AO. (1993). Variability over time of complement activation induced by air bubbles in human and rabbit sera. *J Appl Physiol* 74, 1811-1815.

Bernard F, Bossu JL, Gaillard S. (2001). Identification of living oligodendrocyte developmental stages by fractal analysis of cell morphology. *J Neurosci Res* 65, 439-445.

Bert P, Hitchcock MA, Hitchcock FA. (1943). *Barometric pressure: researches in experimental physiology* (1878). College Book Co., Columbus, Ohio.

Besnard S. (2002). Etude de la distribution et du comportement d'un produit de contraste ultrasonore dans le compartiment vasculaire. Conséquence sur la Physiologie de la plongée sousmarine? Etude théorique de la décompression. In *Médecine Aérospatiale*, pp. 59. Université de Poitiers, Faculté de Medecine et Pharmacie, Poitiers.

Blatteau JE. (1999). Détection des Shunts droite-gauche par echodoppler carotidien: étude versus ETO, à propos de 200 patients. *Medsubhyp* 9, 97-103.

Bogousslavsky J, Garazi S, Jeanrenaud X, Aebischer N, Van Melle G. (1996). *Stroke* recurrence in patients with patent foramen ovale: the Lausanne Study. Lausanne *Stroke* with Paradoxal Embolism Study Group. *Neurology* 46, 1301-1305.

Boussuges A, Blanc F, Carturan D. (2006). Hemodynamic changes induced by recreational scuba diving. *Chest* 129, 1337-1343.

Bove AA. (1998). Risk of decompression sickness with patent foramen ovale. *Undersea Hyperb Med* 25, 175-178.

Boycott AE, Damant GC, Haldane JS. (1908). The prevention of compressed-air ilness. *J Hygiene* 8, 342-443.

Broman T, Branemark PI, Johansson B, Steinwall O. (1966). Intravital and postmortem studies on air embolism damage of the blood-brain barrier tested with trypan blue. *Acta Neurol Scand* 42, 146-152.

Broome JR. (1996). Reduction of decompression illness risk in pigs by use of non-linear ascent profiles. *Undersea Hyperb Med* 23, 19-26.

Brubakk A. (1994). Decompression illness. What we do know, what we don't know. In *First European Consensus Conference on Hyperbaric Medicine, ECHM*, ed. Wattel F, Mathieu D. Université de Lille CRAM.

Brubakk AO. (2003). In *Bennett and Elliott's physiology and medicine of diving*, 5th Ed. Brubakk AO, Neuman TS, pp. xii, 779. Saunders, Edinburgh; New York.

Brubakk AO, Eftedal O. (2001). Comparison of three different ultrasonic methods for quantification of intravascular gas bubbles. *Undersea Hyperb Med* 28, 131-136.

Brubakk AO, Peterson R, Grip A, Holand B, Onarheim J, Segadal K, Kunkle TD, Tonjum S. (1986). Gas bubbles in the circulation of divers after ascending excursions from 300 to 250 msw. *J Appl Physiol* 60, 45-51.

Brubakk AO, Torp H, Angelsen BA. (1991). Noninvasive evaluation of flow changes and gas bubbles in the circulation by combined use of color-flow-imaging and computer postprocessing. *Acta Astronaut* 23, 311-319.

Bryan RN, Cai J, Burke G, Hutchinson RG, Liao D, Toole JF, Dagher AP, Cooper L. (1999). Prevalence and anatomic characteristics of infarct-like lesions on MR images of middle-aged adults: the atherosclerosis risk in communities study. *AJNR Am J Neuroradiol* 20, 1273-1280.

Buhlmann AA. (1975). Decompression theory: Swiss practice. In *Physiology and Medicine of Diving*, 2nd edition edn, ed. Bennet P, Eliott DH, pp. 348-365. Williams and Wilkins, Baltimore.

Bussiere JP, Bonnet D, Renard JL, Monsegu J, Plotton C, Duriez P, De Bourayne J, Ollivier JP. (1992). [Contribution of transesophageal echocardiography in the investigation of the atrium in systemic embolism]. *Ann Med Interne* (Paris) 143, 5-10.

Butler BD. (1996). Cardiopulmonary changes with moderate decompression in rats. National Aeronautics and Space Administration;

National Technical Information Service distributor, Washington, DC, Springfield, VA.

Butler BD, Hills BA. (1979). The lung as a filter for microbubbles. *J Appl Physiol* 47, 537-543.

Buttinelli C, Beccia M, Argentino C. (2002). *Stroke* in a scuba diver with patent foramen ovale. *Eur J Neurol* 9, 89-91.

Byng JW, Boyd NF, Fishell E, Jong RA, Yaffe MJ. (1996a). Automated analysis of mammographic densities. *Phys Med Biol* 41, 909-923.

Byng JW, Boyd NF, Little L, Lockwood G, Fishell E, Jong RA, Yaffe MJ. (1996b). Symmetry of projection in the quantitative analysis of mammographic images. *Eur J Cancer Prev* 5, 319-327.

Cabanes L, Coste J, Derumeaux G, Jeanrenaud X, Lamy C, Zuber M, Mas JL. (2002). Interobserver and intraobserver variability in detection of patent foramen ovale and atrial septal aneurysm with transesophageal echocardiography. *J Am Soc Echocardiogr* 15, 441-446.

Calder IM. (1985). Autopsy and experimental observations on factors leading to barotrauma in man. *Undersea Biomed Res* 12, 165-182.

Calder IM, Sweetnham K, Chan KK, Williams MM. (1987). Relation of alveolar size to forced vital capacity in professional divers. *Br J Ind Med* 44, 467-469.

Caldwell CB, Moran EL, Bogoch ER. (1998). Fractal dimension as a measure of altered trabecular bone in experimental inflammatory arthritis. *J Bone Miner Res* 13, 978-985.

Cambier B. (1993). The anatomophysiology of the atria in adults human hearts. In *Doctoral thesis in Cardiology*, pp. 119. University of Ghent, Ghent.

Cambier B, Vandenbogaerde J, Vakaet L. (1990). Dynamic imaging of the interatrial septum during transesophageal echocardiography and Doppler. *J Anatomy* 173, 246.

Cambier BA, Missault LH, Kockx MM, Vandenbogaerde JF, Alexander JP, Taeymans YM, Van Cauwelaert PA, Brutsaert DL. (1993). Influence of the breathing mode on the time course and amplitude of the cyclic inter-atrial pressure reversal in postoperative coronary bypass surgery patients. *Eur Heart J* 14, 920-924.

Cantais E, Louge P, Suppini A, Foster PP, Palmier B. (2003). Right-to-left shunt and risk of decompression illness with cochleovestibular and cerebral symptoms in divers: case control study in 101 consecutive dive accidents. *Crit Care Med* 31, 84-88.

Carturan D. (1999). Etude de la décompression des plongeurs sportifs: Influence de la vitesse de remontée, de l' âge, de l'aptitude aérobie et de la surcharge pondérale sur la production de bulles intravasculaires circulantes. In *Sciences des Activités Physiques et Sportives*, pp. 88. Université de Méditerranée, Marseille.

Carturan D, Boussuges A, Burnet H, Fondarai J, Vanuxem P, Gardette B. (1999). Circulating venous bubbles in recreational diving: relationships with age, weight, maximal oxygen uptake and body fat percentage. *Int J Sports Med* 20, 410-414.

Carturan D, Boussuges A, Vanuxem P, Bar-Hen A, Burnet H, Gardette B. (2002). Ascent rate, age, maximal oxygen uptake, adiposity, and circulating venous bubbles after diving. *J Appl Physiol* 93, 1349-1356.

Chater N, Brown GD. (1999). Scale-invariance as a unifying psychological principle. *Cognition* 69, B17-24.

Chen WJ, Kuan P, Lien WP, Lin FY. (1992). Detection of patent foramen ovale by contrast trans-esophageal echocardiography. *Chest* 101, 1515-1520.

Chimowitz MI, Nemec JJ, Marwick TH, Lorig RJ, Furlan AJ, Salcedo EE. (1991). Transcranial Doppler ultrasound identifies patients with right-to-left cardiac or pulmonary shunts. *Neurology* 41, 1902-1904.

Chryssanthou C, Springer M, Lipschitz S. (1977). Blood-brain and blood-lung barrier alteration by dysbaric exposure. *Undersea Biomed Res* 4, 117-129.

Cooke JP, Olson RM, Holden RD. (1976). Intravascular bubbles associated with intravenous injections and altitude. *Aviat Space Environ Med* 47, 974-978.

Cordes P, Keil R, Bartsch T, Tetzlaff K, Reuter M, Hutzelmann A, Friege L, Meyer T, Bettinghausen E, Deuschl G. (2000). Neurologic outcome of controlled compressed-air diving. *Neurology* 55, 1743-1745.

Cresswell AG, Grundstrom H, Thorstensson A. (1992). Observations on intra-abdominal pressure and patterns of abdominal intra-muscular activity in man. *Acta Physiol Scand* 144, 409-418.

Crook RA. (1977). Basic medical implications of scuba diving. J Otolaryngol 6, 519-523.

Cross S, S. (1997). *Fractals* in Pathology. *Journal of Pathology* 182, 1-8.

Cross SJ, Evans SA, Thomson LF, Lee HS, Jennings KP, Shields TG. (1992). Safety of subaqua diving with a patent foramen ovale. *BMJ* 304, 481-482.

Cujec B, Mainra R, Johnson DH. (1999). Prevention of recurrent cerebral ischemic events in patients with patent foramen ovale and cryptogenic strokes or transient ischemic attacks. *Can J Cardiol* 15, 57-64.

Cujec B, Polasek P, Mayers I, Johnson D. (1993). Positive end-expiratory pressure increases the right-to-left shunt in mechanically ventilated patients with patent foramen ovale. *Ann Intern Med* 119, 887-894.

Dembert ML. (1977). Scuba diving accidents. *Am Fam Physician* 16, 75-80.

Den Heijer T, Vermeer SE, Clarke R, Oudkerk M, Koudstaal PJ, Hofman A, Breteler MM. (2003). Homocysteine and brain atrophy on MRI of non-demented elderly. *Brain* 126, 170-175.

Di Piero V, Cappagli M, Pastena L, Faralli F, Mainardi G, Di Stani F, Bruti G, Coli A, Lenzi GL, Gagliardi R. (2002). Cerebral effects of hyperbaric oxygen breathing: a CBF SPECT study on professional divers. *Eur J Neurol* 9, 419-421.

Di Tullio M, Sacco RL, Massaro A, Venketasubramanian N, Sherman D, Hoffmann M, Mohr JP, Homma S. (1993a). Transcranial Doppler with contrast injection for the detection of patent foramen ovale in stroke patients. *Int J Card Imaging* 9, 1-5.

Di Tullio M, Sacco RL, Venketasubramanian N, Sherman D, Mohr JP, Homma S. (1993b). Comparison of diagnostic techniques for the detection of a patent foramen ovale in stroke patients. *Stroke* 24, 1020-1024.

Ding J, Nieto FJ, Beauchamp NJ, Longstreth WT, Jr., Manolio TA, Hetmanski JB, Fried LP. (2003). A prospective analysis of risk factors for white matter disease in the brain stem: the Cardiovascular Health Study. *Neuroepidemiology* 22, 275-282.

Dougherty G, Henebry GM. (2002). Lacunarity analysis of spatial pattern in CT images of vertebral trabecular bone for assessing osteoporosis. *Med Eng Phys* 24, 129-138.

Droste DW, Kriete JU, Stypmann J, Castrucci M, Wichter T, Tietje R, Weltermann B, Young P, Ringelstein EB. (1999). Contrast transcranial Doppler ultrasound in the detection of right-to-left shunts: comparison of different procedures and different contrast agents. *Stroke* 30, 1827-1832.

Droste DW, Lakemeier S, Wichter T, Stypmann J, Dittrich R, Ritter M, Moeller M, Freund M, Ringelstein EB. (2002). Optimizing the technique of contrast transcranial Doppler ultrasound in the detection of right-to-left shunts. *Stroke* 33, 2211-2216.

Dujic Z, Duplancic D, Marinovic-Terzic I, Bakovic D, Ivancev V, Valic Z, Eterovic D, Petri NM, Wisloff U, Brubakk AO. (2004). Aerobic exercise before diving reduces venous gas bubble formation in humans. *J Physiol* 555, 637-642.

Dujic Z, Eterovic D, Denoble P, Krstacic G, Tocilj J. (1992). Lung diffusing capacity in a hyperbaric environment: assessment by a rebreathing technique. *Br J Ind Med* 49, 254-259.

Dujic Z, Eterovic D, Denoble P, Krstacic G, Tocilj J, Gosovic S. (1993). Effect of a single air dive on pulmonary diffusing capacity in professional divers. *J Appl Physiol* 74, 55-61.

Eckenhoff RG, Olstad CS, Carrod G. (1990). Human dose-response relationship for decompression and endogenous bubble formation. *J Appl Physiol* 69, 914-918.

Edmonds C, Boughton J. (1985). Intellectual deterioration with excessive diving (punch drunk divers). *Undersea Biomed Res* 12, 321-326.

Edmonds C, Lowry C, Pennefather J. (1992). *Historical and Physiological concepts of decompression. In Diving and Subaquatic Medicine*, ed. Butterworth-Heinemann, pp. 40-158.

Egi SM, Gurmen NM. (2000). Computation of decompression tables using continuous compartment half-lives. *Undersea Hyperb Med* 27, 143-153.

Eke A, Herman P, Bassingthwaighte JB, Raymond GM, Percival DB, Cannon M, Balla I, Ikrenyi C. (2000). Physiological time series: distinguishing fractal noises from motions. *Pflugers Arch* 439, 403-415.

Elliott DH, Hallenbeck JM, Bove AA. (1974a). Acute decompression sickness. *Lancet* 2, 1193-1199.

Elliott DH, Hallenbeck JM, Bove AA. (1974b). Venous infarction of the spinal cord in decompression sickness. *J R Nav Med Serv* 60, 66-71.

Elliott DH, Moon RE. (1993). Manifestation of decompression disorders. In The *Physiology and Medicine of Diving*, ed. Bennet P, Eliott DH, pp. 481-505. Sanders Company Ltd., London.

Evans DE, McDermott JJ, Kobrine AL, Flynn ET. (1988). Effects of intra-venous lidocaine in experimental cerebral air embolism. *Undersea Biomedical Research* 15(supply), 17.

Farkas B, Duboc E, Petrons P, Widelec J, Vanderschueren F, Balestra C, Germonpre P, Marroni A, Cali-Corleo R. (2001). Cerebral lacunary Spots Related To Patency of Foramen Ovale: an MRI Investigation. Preliminary results. In *27 th Annual Meeting, 30 th Anniversary, of The European Underwater and Baromedical Society on Diving and Hyperbaric Medicine*, ed. Van Laak U, pp. 81-82. Geselschaft für Tauch und Überdruckmedizin, Frankfurt, Hanmburg, Germany.

Feltrin GP, Macchi V, Saccavini C, Tosi E, Dus C, Fassina A, Parenti A, De Caro R. (2001). Fractal analysis of lumbar vertebral cancellous bone architecture. *Clin Anat* 14, 414-417.

Ferris E, Engel G. (1951). The Clinical Nature of high altitude decompression sickness. In *Decompression Sickness*, ed. Fulton J. Saunders, London.

Fisher DC, Fisher EA, Budd JH, Rosen SE, Goldman ME. (1995). The incidence of patent foramen ovale in 1,000 consecutive patients. A contrast transesophageal echocardiography study. *Chest* 107, 1504-1509.

Francis TJ, Griffin JL, Homer LD, Pezeshkpour GH, Dutka AJ, Flynn ET. (1990). Bubble-induced dysfunction in acute spinal cord decompression sickness. *J Appl Physiol* 68, 1368-1375.

Francis TJR, Smith DJ. (1991). Describing decompression illness. Undersea Hyperbaric Medical Society.

Freiberger JJ, Denoble PJ, Pieper CF, Uguccioni DM, Pollock NW, Vann RD. (2002). The relative risk of decompression sickness during and after air travel following diving. *Aviat Space Environ Med* 73, 980-984.

Fueredi GA, Czarnecki DJ, Kindwall EP. (1991). MR findings in the brains of compressed-air tunnel workers: relationship to psychometric results. *AJNR Am J Neuroradiol* 12, 67-70.

Fukuda H, Kitani M. (1996). Cigarette smoking is correlated with the periventricular hyperintensity grade of brain magnetic resonance imaging. *Stroke* 27, 645-649.

Gallagher TJ. (1997). Scuba diving accidents: decompression sickness, air embolism. *J Fla Med Assoc* 84, 446-451.

Gardette B. (1979). Correlation between decompression sickness and circulating bubbles in 232 divers. *Undersea Biomed Res* 6, 99-107.

Gardette B. (1989). [Decompression of deep divers]. *Schweiz Z Sportmed* 37, 69-73; discussion 99-102.

Garret JL. (1990). The role of patent foramen ovale in altitude decompression sickness. In *Hypobaric Decompression sickness*, ed. Pilmanis A, pp. 81-92. Brooks Air Base Texas.

Germonpre P. (2005). Patent foramen ovale and diving. *Cardiol Clin* 23, 97-104.

Germonpre P, Balestra C. (2004). Risk of decompression illness among 230 divers in relation to the presence and size of patent foramen ovale. *Eur Heart J* 25, 2173-2174.

Germonpre P, Balestra C, Dendaele P, Unger P, Aerts A, Vanderschueren F, De Pauw M. (1996). Patent Foramen Ovale: a risk factor for cerebral decompression illness in sport divers. In *International Joint Meeting on Hyperbaric Medicine*, ed. Wattel F, Oriani G, Marroni A, pp. 96-99. Galeazzi Hyperbaric Intitute, Milano (Italy).

Germonpre P, Balestra C, Kitoko L, Unger P. (1999). Carotid artery doppler as a minimally invasive screening metrhod for patency of the Foramen Ovale. In *Proceedings of the European Baromedical Society on Diving, Hyperbaric medicine and High Pressure Biology*, ed. Grossman Y, pp. 154-157. Haifa and Eilat (Israel).

Germonpre P, Balestra C, Unger P, Hastier F, Dendaele P. (2002). Time-Related Opening of the foramen ovale in divers. In *28 th Annual Meeting of The European Underwater and Baromedical Society*, ed. P. G, Balestra C. Bruges (Belgium).

Germonpre P, Dendale P, Unger P, Balestra C. (1998a). Patent foramen ovale and decompression sickness in sports divers. *J Appl Physiol* 84, 1622-1626.

Germonpre P, Hastir F, Dendale P, Marroni A, Nguyen AF, Balestra C. (2005). Evidence for increasing patency of the foramen ovale in divers. *Am J Cardiol* 95, 912-915.

Gerriets T, Tetzlaff K, Liceni T, Schafer C, Rosengarten B, Kopiske G, Algermissen C, Struck N, Kaps M. (2000). Arteriovenous bubbles following cold water sport dives: relation to right-to-left shunting. *Neurology* 55, 1741-1743.

Gin K, G., Huckellk V, F., Pollick C. (1993). Femoral vein delivery of contrast medium enhances transthoracic echocardiographic detection of patent foramen ovale. *J Am Coll Cardiol* 22, 1994-1200.

Gotoh Y, Nashimoto I. (1977). [Decompression bubbles in caisson workers (author's transl)]. *Nippon Eiseigaku Zasshi* 32, 529-533.

Greim CA, Trautner H, Kramer K, Zimmermann P, Apfel CC, Roewer N. (2001). The detection of interatrial flow patency in awake and anesthetized patients: a comparative study using transnasal transesophageal echocardiography. *Anesth Analg* 92, 1111-1116.

Groebe G, Marsch WC, Holzmann H. (1990). [The fractals theory and its significance for dermatology]. *Hautarzt* 41, 388-391.

Guyton AC. (1981). Special features of fetal and neonatal physiology. In *Medical Physiology*, ed. Guyton AC, pp. 1037-1046. WB Saunders, Philadelphia.

Ha JW, Shin MS, Kang S, Pyun WB, Jang KJ, Byun KH, Rim SJ, Huh J, Lee BI, Chung N. (2001). Enhanced detection of right-to-left shunt through patent foramen ovale by transthoracic contrast echocardiography using harmonic imaging. *Am J Cardiol* 87, 669-671, A611.

Hagen PT, Scholz DG, Edwards WD. (1984). Incidence and size of patent foramen ovale during the first 10 decades of life: an autopsy study of 965 normal hearts. *Mayo Clin Proc* 59, 17-20.

Hallenbeck JM, Bove AA, Elliott DH. (1975). Mechanisms underlying spinal cord damage in decompression sickness. *Neurology* 25, 308-316.

Hamann GF, Schatzer-Klotz D, Frohlig G, Strittmatter M, Jost V, Berg G, Stopp M, Schimrigk K, Schieffer H. (1998). Femoral injection of echo contrast medium may increase the sensitivity of testing for a patent foramen ovale. *Neurology* 50, 1423-1428.

Handels H, Ross T, Kreusch J, Wolff HH, Poppl SJ. (1998). Image analysis and pattern recognition for computer supported skin tumor diagnosis. *Medinfo* 9 Pt 2, 1056-1062.

Hardy KR. (1997). Diving Related Emergencies. *Emergency Medicine Clinics in North America* 15, 223-240.

Hastings HM, Pekelney R, Monticciolo R, vun Kannon D, del Monte D. (1982). Time scales, persistence and patchiness. *Biosystems* 15, 281-289.

Heckmann JG, Niedermeier W, Brandt-Pohlmann M, Hilz MJ, Hecht M, Neundorfer B. (1999). [Detection of patent foramen ovale. Transesophageal echocardiography and transcranial doppler sonography with ultrasound contrast media are "supplementary, not competing, diagnostic methods"]. *Med Klin* 94, 367-370.

Heier LA, Bauer CJ, Schwartz L, Zimmerman RD, Morgello S, Deck MD. (1989). Large Virchow-Robin spaces: MR-clinical correlation. *AJNR Am J Neuroradiol* 10, 929-936.

Helps SC, Gorman DF. (1991). Air embolism of the brain in rabbits pretreated with mechlorethamine. *Stroke* 22, 351-354.

Hempelman HV. (1993). History of decompression disorders. In The *Physiology and Medicine of Diving*, 4th edition edn, ed. Bennet P, Eliott DH, pp. 342-375. Saunders, London.

Hempleman HV, Florio JT, Garrard MP, Harris DJ, Hayes PA, Hennessy TR, Nichols G, Torok Z, Winsborough MM. (1984). U.K. deep diving trials. *Philos Trans R Soc Lond B Biol Sci* 304, 119-141.

Hennessy TR, Hempleman HV. (1977). An examination of the critical released gas volume concept in decompression sickness. *Proc R Soc Lond B Biol Sci* 197, 299-313.

Heritier F, Schaller MD, Fitting JW, Feihl F, Leuenberger P, Perret C. (1993). [The pulmonary manifestations of diving accidents]. *Schweiz Z Sportmed* 41, 115-120.

Heymans O, Blacher S, Brouers F, Pierard GE. (1999). Fractal quantification of the microvasculature heterogeneity in cutaneous melanoma. *Dermatology* 198, 212-217.

Hierholzer J, Tempka A, Stroszczynski C, Amodio F, Hosten N, Haas J, Felix R. (2000). MRI in decompression illness. *Neuroradiology* 42, 368-370.

Hills BA. (1971). Decompression sickness: a fundamental study of "surface excursion" diving and the selection of limb bends versus C.N.S. symptoms. *Aerosp Med* 42, 833-836.

Hovens MM, ter Riet G, Visser GH. (1995). Long-term adverse effects of scuba diving. *Lancet* 346, 384.

Hsu KJ, Hsu AJ. (1990). Fractal geometry of music. *Proc Natl Acad Sci U S A* 87, 938-941.

Hyldegaard O, Madsen J. (1989). Influence of heliox, oxygen, and N2O-O2 breathing on N2 bubbles in adipose tissue. *Undersea Biomed Res* 16, 185-193.

Hyldegaard O, Madsen J. (1994). Effect of air, heliox, and oxygen breathing on air bubbles in aqueous tissues in the rat. *Undersea Hyperb Med* 21, 413-424.

Hyldegaard O, Moller M, Madsen J. (1991). Effect of He-O2, O2, and N2O-O2 breathing on injected bubbles in spinal white matter. *Undersea Biomed Res* 18, 361-371.

Imbert JP. (1993). Decompression Safety. In *SUBTEC* 93, pp. 238-249. Aberdeen, Scotland.

Imbert JP, Montbaron S. (1990). Use of the Comex Diving Data Base. In *EUBS Workshop on operational dives and decompression data: collection and analysis,* ed. Bakker JA, Sterck J. Amsterdam.

Jauss M, Kaps M, Keberle M, Haberbosch W, Dorndorf W. (1994). A comparison of transesophageal echocardiography and transcranial doppler sonography with contrast medium for detection of patent foramen ovale. *Stroke* 25, 1265-1267.

Job FP, Ringelstein EB, Grafen Y, Flachskampf FA, Doherty C, Stockmanns A, Hanrath P. (1994). Comparison of transcranial contrast doppler sonography and transesophageal contrast echocardiography for the detection of patent foramen ovale in young stroke patients. *Am J Cardiol* 74, 381-384.

Jungreis CA, Kanal E, Hirsch WL, Martinez AJ, Moossy J. (1988). Normal perivascular spaces mimicking lacunar infarction: MR imaging. *Radiology* 169, 101-104.

Kampen J, Koch A, Struck N. (2001). Methodological remarks on transcranial doppler ultrasonography for PFO detection. *Anesthesiology* 95, 808-809.

Keipes M, Ries F, Dicato M. (1993). Of the British coastline and the interest of fractals in medicine. *Biomed Pharmacother* 47, 409-415.

Kelemen G. (1983). Temporal bone findings in cases of salt water drowning. *Ann Otol Rhinol Laryngol* 92, 134-136.

Kelleher PC, Pethybridge RJ, Francis TJ. (1996). Outcome of neurological decompression illness: development of a manifestation-based model. *Aviat Space Environ Med* 67, 654-658.

Kilgore KS, Friedrichs GS, Homeister JW, Lucchesi BR. (1994). The complement system in myocardial ischaemia/reperfusion injury. *Cardiovasc Res* 28, 437-444.

Kindwall EP. (1998). Compressed air work. In The *Physiology and Medicine of Diving*, ed. Bennet P, Elliott DS, pp. 1-18. W B Saunders Company Ltd., London.

Klinkner DB, Densmore JC, Kaul S, Noll L, Lim HJ, Weihrauch D, Pritchard KA, Jr., Oldham KT, Sander TL. (2006). Endothelium-derived microparticles inhibit human cardiac valve endothelial cell function. *Shock* 25, 575-580.

Klotzsch C, Janssen G, Berlit P. (1994). Transesophageal echocardiography and contrast-TCD in the detection of a patent foramen ovale: experiences with 111 patients. *Neurology* 44, 1603-1606.

Knauth M, Ries S, Pohimann S, Kerby T, Forsting M, Daffertshofer M, Hennerici M, Sartor K. (1997). Cohort study of multiple brain lesions in sport divers: role of a patent foramen ovale. *Bmj* 314, 701-705.

Kumar KV, Waligora JM, Calkins DS. (1990). Threshold altitude resulting in decompression sickness. *Aviat Space Environ Med* 61, 685-689.

Lamy C, Giannesini C, Zuber M, Arquizan C, Meder JF, Trystram D, Coste J, Mas JL. (2002a). Clinical and Imaging Findings in Cryptogenic Stroke Patients With and Without Patent Foramen Ovale: The PFO-ASA Study. *Stroke* 33, 706-711.

Lamy C, Giannesini C, Zuber M, Arquizan C, Meder JF, Trystram D, Coste J, Mas JL. (2002b). Clinical and imaging findings in cryptogenic stroke patients with and without patent foramen ovale: the PFO-ASA Study. Atrial Septal Aneurysm. *Stroke* 33, 706-711.

Landini G. (1997). Is periodontal breakdown a fractal process? Simulations using the Weierstrass-Mandelbrot function. *J Periodontal Res* 32, 300-307.

Landsberg PG. (1976). South African underwater diving accidents, 1969-1976. *S Afr Med J* 50, 2155-2159.

Laupacis A, Sackett DL, Roberts RS. (1988). An assessment of clinically useful measures of the consequences of treatment. *N Engl J Med* 318, 1728-1733.

Lechat P, Lascault G, Mas JL, Loron P, Klimczac K, Guggiari M, Drobinski G, Fraysse JB, Thomas D, Grosgogeat Y. (1989). [Prevalence of patent foramen ovale in young patients with ischemic cerebral complications]. *Arch Mal Coeur Vaiss* 82, 847-852.

Lechner H, Schmidt R, Bertha G, Justich E, Offenbacher H, Schneider G. (1988). Nuclear magnetic resonance image white matter lesions and risk factors for stroke in normal individuals. *Stroke* 19, 263-265.

Lee J, Matthews MB, Sharpey-Schafer EP. (1954). The effect of the valsalva maneuver on the systemic and pulmonary arterial pressure in man. *St Thomas Hospital Bulletin* Apr., 311-316.

Leitch DR. (1985). Complications of saturation diving. *J R Soc Med* 78, 634-637.

Leitch DR, Barnard EE. (1982). Observations on no-stop and repetitive air and oxynitrogen diving. *Undersea Biomed Res* 9, 113-129.

Lespessailles E, Poupon S, Niamane R, Loiseau-Peres S, Derommelaere G, Harba R, Courteix D, Benhamou CL. (2002). Fractal analysis of trabecular bone texture on calcaneus radiographs: effects of age, time since menopause and hormone replacement therapy. *Osteoporos Int* 13, 366-372.

Libouban H, Moreau MF, Legrand E, Audran M, Basle MF, Chappard D. (2002). Comparison of histomorphometric descriptors of bone architecture with dual-energy X-ray absorptiometry for assessing bone loss in the orchidectomized rat. *Osteoporos Int* 13, 422-428.

Losa GA, Nonnenmacher TF. (1996). Self-similarity and fractal irregularity in pathologic tissues. *Mod Pathol* 9, 174-182.

Lutz J, Herrmann G. (1984). Perfluorochemicals as a treatment of decompression sickness in rats. *Pflugers Arch* 401, 174-177.

Luzi P, Bianciardi G, Miracco C, De Santi MM, Del Vecchio MT, Alia L, Tosi P. (1999). Fractal analysis in human pathology. *Ann N Y Acad Sci* 879, 255-257.

Maier T. (1998). [Chaos theory and complexity in psychiatry]. *Psychother Psychosom Med Psychol* 48, 314-317.

Mandelbrot BB. (1983). *The fractal geometry of nature*. W.H. Freeman, San Francisco.

Mandelbrot BB, Kol B, Aharony A. (2002). Angular gaps in radial diffusion-limited aggregation: two fractal dimensions and nontransient deviations from linear self-similarity. *Phys Rev Lett* 88, 055501.

Marroni A, Balestra C. (1996). DAN Oxygen First Aid in Dive Accidents, pp. 70. DAN Europe (Anglais).

Marroni A, Bennett P, B., Balestra C, Cali-Corleo R, Germonpre P, Pieri M, Bonuccelli C. (2002a). What Ascent Profile for the Prevention of Decompression Sickness? 2 - A field model comparing hill and haldane ascent modalities, with an eye to the development of a bubble decompression algorithm. In *28 th Annual Scientific Meeting of The European Underwater and Baromedical Society*, ed. Germonpre P, Balestra C, pp. 44-48. ACHOBEL Brussels, Belgium 2002, Brugge, Belgium.

Marroni A, Bennett P, Balestra C, Cali Corleo R, Germonpré P, Pieri M, Bonucelli C. (2002b). What ascent profile for the prevention of decompression sickness? II - A field model comparing hill and haldane ascent modalities, with an eye to de development of a bubble-safe decompression algorythm. DAN Europe DSL Special Project "Haldane Vs Hill". *European Journal of Underwater and Hyperbaric Medicine* 3, 75.

Marroni A, Bennett P, Cronjé FJ, Cali Corleo R, Germonpre P, Pieri M, Bonuccelli C, Balestra C. (2004a). A deep stop during decompression from 82 fsw (25 m) significantly reduces bubbles and fast tissue gas tensions. *Undersea Hyperb Med* 31, 233-243.

Marroni A, Bennett PB, Cronjé FJ, Germonpre P, Pieri M, Bonuccelli C, Balestra C. (2004b). comparison of precordial doppler detected bubbles and computer measured gas tensions in dives to 25m with linear ascents, deep and shallow stops. *Undersea Hyperb Med* 31, (In Press).

Marroni A, Cali-Corleo R, Balestra C, Longobardi P, Germonpre P, Voellm E, Pieri M, Pepoli R. (2001a). Incidence of asymptomatic ciculating venous gas emboli in unrestricted, uneventful recreational diving. Skin cooling appears to be related to post dive doppler detectable bubble production. An unexpected finding. DSL Special Project 03-2001. In *27 th Annual Meeting, 30 th Anniversary, of The European Underwater and Baromedical Society on Diving and Hyperbaric Medicine*, ed. Van Laak U, pp. 79-80. Gesellschaft für Tauch und Überdruckmedizin, Frankfurt, Hanmburg, Germany.

Marroni A, Cali-Corleo R, Balestra C, Longobardi P, Germonpre P, Voellm E, Pieri M, Pepoli R. (2001b). The speed of ascent dilemma: "instant speed of ascent" or "time to surface" - Which one really matters? Instant speed of ascent vs. delta-p in The leading tissue and post-dive doppler bubble production. DSL Special Project 02/2001. In *27 th Annual Meeting, 30 th Anniversary, of The European Underwater and Baromedical Society on Diving and Hyperbaric Medicine*, ed. Van Laak U, pp. 74-78. Gesellschaft für Tauch und Überdruckmedizin, Frankfurt, Hanmburg, Germany.

Marroni A, Cali-Corleo R, Balestra C, Longobardi P, Germonpre P, Voellm E, Pieri M, Pepoli R. (2001c). The Use of a "Proportional M value Reduction Concepr" (PMRC) Changing the ascent profile with de intoduction of extra deep stops reduces the production of circulating venous gas emboli after compressed air diving. DSL Special Project. In *27 th Annual Meeting, 30 th Anniversary, of The European Underwater and Baromedical Society on Diving and Hyperbaric Medicine*, ed. Van Laak U, pp. 69-73. Gesellschaft für Tauch und Überdruckmedizin, Frankfurt, Hanmburg, Germany.

Marroni A, Cali-Corleo R, Balestra C, Voellm E, Pieri M. (2000). Incidence of asymptomatic circulating venous gas emboli in unrestricted uneventful recreational diving. DAN europe safe dive first results. In *24 th Annual Scientific Meeting of The European Underwater and Baromedical Society*, ed. Cali-Corleo R, pp. 9-15. EUBS, Valletta, Malta.

Marroni A, Cali Corleo R, Denoble P. (1996). Understanding the safety of recreational div-ing. DAN Europe's Project SAFE DIVE Phase I: fine tuning of the field research engine and methods. In *International Joint Meeting on Hyperbaric and Underwater Medicine, EUBS, ECHM, ICHM, DAN*, ed. Wattel F, Marroni A, pp. 279-284. Minerva, Milano (Istituto Galeazzi).

Marroni A, Zannini D. (1981). [Effects of variations in the ascending speed on the production of circulating gas bubbles after compressed-air diving]. *Minerva Med* 72, 3567-3572.

Marroni A, Zannini D, Marcenaro A. (1983). [Physiopathologic changes and morbidity in divers in satu-ration. Epidemiologic evaluation of 9 years' activities (1973-1982)]. *Minerva Med* 74, 2015-2021.

Martin SE, Chenoweth DE, Engler RL, Roth DM, Longhurst JC. (1988). C5a decreases regional coronary blood flow and myocardial function in pigs: implications for a granulocyte mecha-nism. *Circ Res* 63, 483-491.

Martini S, Brubakk AO, Bech C. (1989). Effect of high pressure on metabolic response to cold in rats. *Acta Physiol Scand* 135, 359-366.

Mas J-L, Arquizan C, Lamy C, Zuber M, Cabanes L, Derumeaux G, Coste J. The patent foramen ovale and atrial septal aneurysm study group. (2001). Recurrent cerebrovascular events associated with patent foramen ovale, atrial septal aneurysm, or both. *N Engl J Med* 345, 1740-1746.

McQueen D, Kent G, Murrison A. (1994). Self-reported long-term effects of diving and decom-pression illness in recreational scuba divers. *Br J Sports Med* 28, 101-104.

Meisel LV. (1992). Generalized Mandelbrot rule for fractal sections. *Physical Review* A 45, 654-656.

Michalodimitrakis E, Patsalis A. (1987). Nitrogen narcosis and alcohol consumption—a scuba div-ing fatality. *J Forensic Sci* 32, 1095-1097.

Michiels K. (1999). Neurotoxiceit ten gevolde van solvenbloodstelling een onderzoek de predic-tive waarde van verwijscriteria op basis van de resultaten van het Neurosreen test program-ma. In *Neuropsychology department AZ Leuven*, pp. 89. Katholiek Universiteit van Leuven, Leuven.

Miller JN, Fagraeus L, Bennett PB, Elliott DH, Shields TG, Grimstad J. (1978). Nitrogen-oxygen satu-ration therapy in serious cases of compressed-air decompression sickness. *Lancet* 2, 169-171.

Mitchell SJ. (2001). Lidocaine in the treatment of decompression illness: a review of the litera-ture. *Undersea Hyperb Med* 28, 165-174.

Moir EW. (1896). Tunneling by Compressed air. *Journal of the Society of Arts* 44, 567.

Moon RE, Camporesi EM, Kisslo JA. (1989). Patent foramen ovale and decompression sickness in divers. *Lancet* 1, 513-514.

Moore L, Bignold LP. (1988). Generalised angiosarcoma of the heart. *Virchows Arch A Pathol Anat Histopathol* 413, 87-90.

Morel O, Toti F, Bakouboula B, Grunebaum L, Freyssinet JM. (2006a). Procoagulant microparti-cles: 'criminal partners' in atherothrombosis and deleterious cellular exchanges. *Pathophysiol Haemost Thromb* 35, 15-22.

Morel O, Toti F, Hugel B, Bakouboula B, Camoin-Jau L, Dignat-George F, Freyssinet JM. (2006b). Procoagulant microparticles: disrupting the vascular homeostasis equation? *Arterioscler Thromb Vasc Biol* 26, 2594-2604.

Morgan WP. (1995). Anxiety and panic in recreational scuba divers. *Sports Med* 20, 398-421.

Morild I, Mork SJ. (1994). A neuropathologic study of the ependymoventricular surface in diver brains. *Undersea Hyperb Med* 21, 43-51.

Mork SJ, Morild I, Brubakk AO, Eidsvik S, Nyland H. (1994). A histopathologic and immunocy-tochemical study of the spinal cord in amateur and professional divers. *Undersea Hyperb Med* 21, 391-402.

Motulsky H. (1995). *Intuitive Biostatistics*. Oxford University Press, New York.

Murrison AW, Lacey EJ, Restler M, Martinique J, Francis TJ. (1991). Ten years of diving-related illness in the Royal Navy. *J Soc Occup Med* 41, 89-93.

Nadas AS, Fyler DC. (1972). Communications between systemic and pulmonary circuits with predominantly left-to-right shunts. In *Pediatric Cardiology*, ed. Nadas AS, Fyler DC, pp. 317-452. WB Saunders, Philadelphia.

Nishi R. (1993). Doppler and ultrasonic bubble detection. In The *Physiology and Medicine of Diving*, ed. Bennett P, Elliott DH, pp. 433-453. W.B. Saunders, London, UK.

Nygren AT, Jogestrand T. (1998). Detection of patent foramen ovale by transcranial Doppler and carotid duplex ultrasonography: a comparison with transoesophageal echocardiography. *Clin Physiol* 18, 327-330.

O'Leary DS, Block RI, Koeppel JA, Flaum M, Schultz SK, Andreasen NC, Ponto LB, Watkins GL, Hurtig RR, Hichwa RD. (2002). Effects of smoking marijuana on brain perfusion and cognition. *Neuropsychopharmacology* 26, 802-816.

Palmer AC, Calder IM, Hughes JT. (1987). Spinal cord degeneration in divers. *Lancet* 2, 1365-1366.

Palmer AC, Calder IM, Yates PO. (1992). *Cerebral Vasculopathy in Divers. Neuropath and Appl Neurobiol* 18, 113-124.

Patten BM. (1931). The closure of the Foramen ovale. *Am J Anat* 48, 19-44.

Patten BM. (1953). Postnatal changes in Circulation. In *Human Embryology*, ed. Patten BM, pp. 691-705. Mc Graw-Hill Book Company, New York.

Paumgartner D, Losa G, Weibel ER. (1981). Resolution effect on the stereological estimation of surface and volume and its interpretation in terms of fractal dimensions. *J Microsc* 121, 51-63.

Peyrin E, Guillaume YC. (1999). Reanalysis of solute retention on immobilized human serum albumin using fractal geometry. *Anal Chem* 71, 1496-1499.

Pfleger S, Konstantin Haase K, Stark S, Latsch A, Simonis B, Scherhag A, Schumacher, Voelker W, Borggrefe M. (2001). Haemodynamic quantification of different provocation manoeuvres by simultaneous measurement of right and left atrial pressure: implications for the echocardiographic detection of persistent foramen ovale. *Eur J Echocardiogr* 2, 88-93.

Piccin A, Murphy WG, Smith OP. (2006). Circulating microparticles: pathophysiology and clinical implications. *Blood Rev.*

Pol M, Wattelle M. (1854). Mémoire sur les effets de la compression de l'air appliquée au creusement des puits à Houille. *Annales d'hygiene publique et de médecine légale* Second series, 241.

Pollard GW, Marsh PL, Fife CE, Smith LR, Vann RD. (1995). Ascent rate, post-dive exercise, and decompression sickness in the rat. *Undersea Hyperb Med* 22, 367-376.

Porter R, Ghosh S, Lange GD, Smith TG, Jr. (1991). A fractal analysis of pyramidal neurons in mammalian motor cortex. *Neurosci Lett* 130, 112-116.

Pyle R. (1999). The importance of deep diving stops: rethinking ascent patterns from decompression dives. In *Deep Tech*, pp. 64-65.

Reul J, Weis J, Jung A, Willmes K, Thron A. (1995). Central nervous system lesions and cervical disc herniations in amateur divers. *Lancet* 345, 1403-1405.

Reuter M, Tetzlaff K, Hutzelmann A, Fritsch G, Steffens JC, Bettinghausen E, Heller M. (1997). MR imaging of the central nervous system in diving-related decompression illness. *Acta Radiol* 38, 940-944.

Rigaut JP, Schoevaert-Brossault D, Downs AM, Landini G. (1998). Asymptotic fractals in the context of grey-scale images. *J Microsc* 189 (Pt 1), 57-63.

Rinck PA, Svihus R, de Francisco P. (1991). MR imaging of the central nervous system in divers. *J Magn Reson Imaging* 1, 293-299.

Rogers G. (1995). Long-term adverse effects of scuba diving. *Lancet* 346, 385.

Rohr Lefloch J. (1994). Patent foramen ovale and paradoxical embolism. *Rev Neurol* 150, 282-285.

Rossitti S. (1995). Energetic and spatial constraints of arterial networks. *Arq Neuropsiquiatr* 53, 333-341.

Rouvière H, Delmas A. (1985). *Anatomie Humaine,* vol. 2 Tronc. Masson, Paris.

Saary MJ, Gray GW. (2001). A review of the relationship between patent foramen ovale and type II decompression sickness. *Aviat Space Environ Med* 72, 1113-1120.

Sacco RL, Homma S, Di Tullio MR. (1993). Patent foramen ovale: a new risk factor for ischemic stroke. Heart Dis *Stroke* 2, 235-241.

Sadler C. (1990a). A child's living hell. *Nurs Times* 86, 19.

Sadler TW. (1990b). Cardiovascular System. In *Langman's Medical Embryology*, ed. Sadler TW.

Sadler TW, Langman J. (2000). *Langman's medical embryology*. Lippincott Williams, Wilkins, Philadelphia.

Sadler TW, Langman J. (2004). *Langman's medical embryology*. Lippincott Williams, Wilkins, Philadelphia.

Schellart NA. (1992). Contrast sensitivity of air-breathing nonprofessional scuba divers at a depth of 40 meters. *Percept Mot Skills* 75, 275-283.

Schindler J. (1993). Dynamics of Bacillus colony growth. *Trends Microbiol* 1, 333-338.

Schneider B, Zienkiewicz T, Jansen V, Hofmann T, Noltenius H, Meinertz T. (1996). Diagnosis of patent foramen ovale by transesophageal echocardiography and correlation with autopsy findings. *Am J Cardiol* 77, 1202-1209.

Schuchlenz HW, Weihs W, Beitzke A, Stein J-I, Gamillscheg A, Rehak P. (2002a). Transesophageal Echocardiography for Quantifying Size of Patent Foramen Ovale in Patients With Cryptogenic Cerebrovascular Events. *Stroke* 33, 293-296.

Schuchlenz HW, Weihs W, Beitzke A, Stein JI, Gamillscheg A, Rehak P. (2002b). Transesophageal echocardiography for quantifying size of patent foramen ovale in patients with cryptogenic cerebrovascular events. *Stroke* 33, 293-296.

Schuchlenz HW, Weihs W, Horner S, Quehenberger F. (2000). The Association Between tha Diameter of a Patent Foramen Ovale and the Risk of Embolic Cerebrovascular Events. *Am J Med* 109, 456-462.

Schwerzmann M, Seiler C. (2001). Recreational scuba diving, patent foramen ovale and their associated risks. *Swiss Med Wkly* 131, 365-374.

Shinoda S, Hasegawa Y, Kawasaki S, Tagawa N, Iwata H. (1997). Magnetic resonance imaging of osteonecrosis in divers: comparison with plain radiographs. *Skeletal Radiol* 26, 354-359.

Simak J, Gelderman MP, Yu H, Wright V, Baird AE. (2006). Circulating endothelial microparticles in acute ischemic stroke: a link to severity, lesion volume and outcome. *J Thromb Haemost* 4, 1296-1302.

Siostrzonek P, Zangeneh M, Gossinger H, Lang W, Rosenmayr G, Heinz G, Stumpflen A, Zeiler K, Schwarz M, Mosslacher H. (1991). Comparison of transesophageal and transthoracic contrast echocardiography for detection of a patent foramen ovale. *Am J Cardiol* 68, 1247-1249.

Sisodiya SM, Free SL, Fish DR, Shorvon SD. (1995). Increasing the yield from volumetric MRI in patients with epilepsy. *Magn Reson Imaging* 13, 1147-1152.

Slosman DO, De Ribaupierre S, Chicherio C, Ludwig C, Montandon ML, Allaoua M, Genton L, Pichard C, Grousset A, Mayer E, Annoni JM, De Ribaupierre A. (2004). Negative neurofunctional effects of frequency, depth and environment in recreational scuba diving: the Geneva "memory dive" study. *Br J Sports Med* 38, 108-114.

Smith DJ, Francis TJ, Hodgson M, Murrison AW, Sykes JJ. (1990a). Interatrial shunts and decompression sickness in divers. *Lancet* 335, 1593.

Smith DJ, Francis TJ, Hodgson M, Murrison AW, Sykes JJ. (1990b). Interatrial shunts and decompression sickness in divers. *Lancet* 335, 914-915.

Sparacia G, Banco A, Sparacia B, Midiri M, Brancatelli G, Accardi M, Lagalla R. (1997). Magnetic resonance findings in scuba diving-related spinal cord decompression sickness. *Magma* 5, 111-115.

Spencer MP, Johanson DC. (1974). Investigation of new principles for human decompression schedules using the Doppler ultrasonic blood bubble detector. Institute for Environmental Medicine and Physiology, Seattle, Washington. USA.

Steinbruck K, Paeslack V. (1980). Analysis of 139 spinal cord injuries due to accidents in water sports. *Paraplegia* 18, 86-93.

Stevens DM, Gartner SL, Pearson RR, Flynn ET, Mink RB, Robinson DH, Dutka AJ. (1993). Complement activation during saturation diving. *Undersea Hyperb Med* 20, 279-288.

Stoddard MF, Keedy DL, Dawkins PR. (1993). The cough test is superior to the valsalva maneuver in the delineation of right-to-left shunting through a patent foramen ovale during contrast transesophageal echocardiography. *Am Heart J* 125, 185-189.

Strunk BL, Cheitlin MD, Stulbarg MS, Schiller NB. (1987). Right-to-left interatrial shunting through a patent foramen ovale despite normal intracardiac pressures. *Am J Cardiol* 60, 413-415.

Swerlick RA, Yancey KB, Lawley TJ. (1988). A direct in vivo comparison of the inflammatory properties of human C5a and C5a des Arg in human skin. *J Immunol* 140, 2376-2381.

Sztajzel R, Genoud D, Roth S, Mermillod B, Le Floch-Rohr J. (2002). Patent foramen ovale, a possible cause of symptomatic migraine: a study of 74 patients with acute ischemic stroke. *Cerebrovasc Dis* 13, 102-106.

Takahashi T, Murata T, Omori M, Kimura H, Kado H, Kosaka H, Takahashi K, Itoh H, Wada Y. (2001). Quantitative evaluation of magnetic resonance imaging of deep white matter hyperintensity in geriatric patients by multifractal analysis. *Neurosci Lett* 314, 143-146.

Taylor WD, MacFall JR, Steffens DC, Payne ME, Provenzale JM, Krishnan KR. (2003). Localization of age-associated white matter hyperintensities in late-life depression. Prog Neuropsychopharmacol *Biol Psychiatry* 27, 539-544.

Testut L, Latarjet A. (1948). *Traité d'Anatomie Humaine*. Dion, Paris.

Tetzlaff K, Friege L, Hutzelmann A, Reuter M, Holl D, Leplow B. (1999). Magnetic resonance signal abnormalities and neuropsychological deficits in elderly compressed-air divers. *Eur Neurol* 42, 194-199.

Thill A, Veerapaneni S, Simon B, Wiesner M, Bottero JY, Snidaro D. (1998). Determination of structure of aggregates by confocal scanning laser microscopy. *J Colloid Interface Sci* 204, 357-362.

Thompson-Schill SL, Jonides J, Marshuetz C, Smith EE, D'Esposito M, Kan IP, Knight RT, Swick D. (2002). Effects of frontal lobe damage on interference effects in working memory. *Cogn Affect Behav Neurosci* 2, 109-120.

Thorsen T, Brubakk A, Ovstedal T, Farstad M, Holmsen H. (1986). A method for production of N2 microbubbles in platelet-rich plasma in an aggregometer-like apparatus, and effect on the platelet density in vitro. *Undersea Biomed Res* 13, 271-288.

Todnem K, Nyland H, Skeidsvoll H, Svihus R, Rinck P, Kambestad BK, Riise T, Aarli JA. (1991). Neurological long term consequences of deep diving. *Br J Ind Med* 48, 258-266.

Torti SR, Billinger M, Schwerzmann M, Vogel R, Zbinden R, Windecker S, Seiler C. (2004). Risk of decompression illness among 230 divers in relation to the presence and size of patent foramen ovale. *Eur Heart J* 25, 1014-1020.

Trefousse C, Vallee J-F. (1991). Fractales Une géométrie de la nature une géométrie du chaos. France,FR3,Zeaux Productions,RTBF.

Triger M. (1845). Letter to Monsieur Arago. In Comptes rendus De l'Académie des Sciences, pp. 445-449. Paris.

Tsai LM, Chen JH. (1990). Abnormal hemodynamic response to valsalva maneuver in patients with atrial septal defect evaluated by doppler echocardiography. *Chest* 98, 1175-1178.

Uguccioni D, Vann RD, Smith LR, Butler BD, Roye BD, Roer RD. (1995). Effect of safety stops on venous gas emboli after no stop diving. *Undersea & Hyperbaric Medicine*, 38-39.

Valentine R. (2000). Physiologists, Fathometers and Menfish. In *10th Conference Historical Diving Society*, pp. 10-14. Historical Diving Times, Plymouth UK.

Van Camp G, Cosynns B, Vandenbossche J-L. (1994). Non smoke spontaneouscontrast in left atrium intensified by respiratory manoeuvres: a new transesophageal echocardiographic observation. *Br Heart J* 72, 446-451.

Van Camp G, Schulze D, Cosyns B, Vandenbossche JL. (1993). Relation between patent foramen ovale and unexplained stroke. *Am J Cardiol* 71, 596-598.

Van Der Aue OE, White WA, Hayter R, Brinton FS, Kellar RJ, Behnke AR. (1945). Physiological factors underlying the prevention and treatment of decompression sickness. USN Experimental Diving Unit, Washington, D.C.

Van Dijk EJ, Prins ND, Vermeer SE, Koudstaal PJ, Breteler MM. (2002). Frequency of white matter lesions and silent lacunar infarcts. *J Neural Transm Suppl*, 25-39.

Vandenbogaerde J, De Bleecker J, Decoo D, Francois K, Cambier B, Bergen JM, Vandermersch C, De Reuck J, Clement DL. (1992). Transoesophageal echo-doppler in patients suspected of a cardiac source of peripheral emboli. *Eur Heart J* 13, 88-94.

Vann RD, Denoble P, Emmerman MN, Corson KS. (1993). Flying after diving and decompression sickness. *Aviat Space Environ Med* 64, 801-807.

Velanovich V. (1998). Fractal analysis of mammographic lesions: a prospective, blinded trial. *Breast Cancer Res Treat* 49, 245-249.

Vermeer SE, Prins ND, den Heijer T, Hofman A, Koudstaal PJ, Breteler MM. (2003). Silent brain infarcts and the risk of dementia and cognitive decline. *N Engl J Med* 348, 1215-1222.

Versprille A, Jansen JR, Scheuder JJ. (1982). Dynamic aspects of interaction between airway pressure and the circulation. In *Applied physiology in clinical respiratory care*, ed. Prakash O, pp. 447-463. Martinus Nijhoff, Den Hague.

Vik A, Brubakk AO, Hennessy TR, Jenssen BM, Ekker M, Slordahl SA. (1990). Venous air embolism in swine: transport of gas bubbles through the pulmonary circulation. *J Appl Physiol* 69, 237-244.

Vik A, Jenssen BM, Brubakk AO. (1992). Paradoxical air embolism in pigs with a patent foramen ovale. *Undersea Biomed Res* 19, 361-374.

Vik A, Jenssen BM, Brubakk AO. (1993). Arterial gas bubbles after decompression in pigs with patent foramen ovale. *Undersea Hyperb Med* 20, 121-131.

Wahl A, Windecker S, Meier B. (2001). Patent foramen ovale: pathophysiology and therapeutic options in symptomatic patients. *Minerva Cardioangiol* 49, 403-411.

Waligora JM, Horrigan DJ, Jr., Conkin J. (1987). The effect of extended O2 prebreathing on altitude decompression sickness and venous gas bubbles. *Aviat Space Environ Med* 58, A110-112.

Waligora JM, Horrigan DJ, Nicogossian A. (1991). The physiology of spacecraft and space suit atmosphere selection. *Acta Astronaut* 23, 171-177.

Ward CL. (1967). Scuba diving—biologic and physical aspects. Review 1-67. *Aeromed Rev* 1, 1-25.

Ward R, Jones D, Haponik EF. (1995). Paradoxical embolism. An underrecognized problem. *Chest* 108, 549-558.

Webb J, Engel G, Romano J. (1944a). The mechanism of pain in aviators: "Bends". *J Clin Invest* 23, 934-935.

Webb J, Ferris E, Engel G. (1944b). Radiographic studies of the knee during bends, pp. 305. US NRC Comm Aviat Med report, Washington.

Wilmshurst P. (1997). Brain Damage in Divers. *British Medical Journal* 314, 689-690.

Wilmshurst P, Allen C, Parish T. (1994). Incidence of decompression illness in amateur scuba divers. *Health Trends* 26, 116-118.

Wilmshurst P, Edge CJ, Bryson P. (1995). Long-term adverse effects of scuba diving. *Lancet* 346, 384.

Wilmshurst P, Ross K. (1998). Dysbaric osteonecrosis of the shoulder in a sport scuba diver. *Br J Sports Med* 32, 344-345.

Wilmshurst PT, Ellis BG, Jenkins BS. (1986). Paradoxical gas embolism in a scuba diver with an atrial septal defect. *Br Med J* (Clin Res Ed) 293, 1277.

Wilmshurst PT, Nuri M, Crowther A, Webb-Peploe MM. (1989). Cold-induced pulmonary oedema in scuba divers and swimmers and subsequent development of hypertension. *Lancet* 1, 62-65.

Wisloff U, Brubakk AO. (2001). Aerobic endurance training reduces bubble formation and increases survival in rats exposed to hyperbaric pressure. *J Physiol* 537, 607-611.

Wisloff U, Richardson RS, Brubakk AO. (2003). NOS inhibition increases bubble formation and reduces survival in sedentary but not exercised rats. *J Physiol* 546, 577-582.

Wisloff U, Richardson RS, Brubakk AO. (2004). Exercise and nitric oxide prevent bubble formation: a novel approach to the prevention of decompression sickness? *J Physiol* 555, 825-829.

Wong RM. (2003). Empirical Diving Techniques. In *Bennett and Eliott's Physiology and Medicine of Diving*, 5th edn, ed. Brubakk A, Neuman TO, pp. 64-76. Saunders, London.

Workman R. (1965). Calculation of decompression schedules for nitrogen-oxygen and helium-oxygen dives. U.S. Navy Experimental Diving Unit, Washington.

Yamashita K, Kobayashi S, Yamaguchi S, Koide H. (1996). Cigarette smoking and silent brain infarction in normal adults. *Intern Med* 35, 704-706.

Yanagawa Y, Okada Y, Terai C, Ikeda T, Ishida K, Fukuda H, Hirata F, Fujita K. (1998). MR imaging of the central nervous system in divers. *Aviat Space Environ Med* 69, 892-895.

Yarbrough OD, Behnke AR. (1939). The treatment of compressed air illness utilising oxygen. *J Ind Hyg Toxicol* 21, 213-218.

Yetkin E, Ozisik II, Ozcan C, Aksoy Y, Turhan H. (2006). Decreased endothelium-dependent vasodilatation in patients with migraine: a new aspect to vascular pathophysiology of migraine. *Coron Artery Dis* 17, 29-33.

Zasslow MA, Pearl RG, Larson CP, Silverberg G, Shuer LF. (1988). PEEP does not affect left atrial-right atrial pressure difference in neurosurgical patients. *Anesthesiology* 68, 760-763.

Zheng L, Chan AK. (2001). An artificial intelligent algorithm for tumor detection in screening mammogram. *IEEE Trans Med Imaging* 20, 559-567.

NOTES